Exercising and Loving It

Your Simple Lazy Way to Get Fit and Great Shape

I0089616

Coach Jim Everroad
National Fitness Hall of Fame Inductee
Two Million Copies Sold

Trius Publishing
San Diego, CA
republished 2022 in conjuction with
Everroad Publishing Company
Columbus, IN
2012

Exercising and Loving It

Copyright© 2012 by James M. Everroad
Published by Everroad Publishing Company
Columbus, IN 47201

Paperback first edition ISBN: 978-0-9674594-2-4

Library of Congress Control Number: 2012920156

Printed in the United States of America

Reprinted by Trius Publishing
San Diego, CA 92119
in conjunction with
Everroad Publishing Company
2022

The author of this book does not dispense medical advice or prescribe the use of any technique as a form of treatment for physical or mental problems without the advice of a physician, either directly or indirectly. The intent of the author is only to offer information of a general nature to help you in your quest for performance improvement. In the event you use any of the information in this book for yourself or to help others is your constitutional right, the author and publishers assume no responsibility for your actions.

Second Edition Paperback   ISBN: 978-0-9986357-8-1
Second Edition E-book .epub ISBN: 978-1-961817-17-3

CONTENTS

DEDICATION   5
ACKNOWLEDGEMENTS   6
PREFACE   7

PART ONE
YOUR LAZY WAY TO GREAT SHAPE

YOUR LAZY WAY TO GREAT SHAPE?   13
HEALTH AND FITNESS BENEFITS   15
WHY YOUR LAZY WAY TO GREAT SHAPE WORKS   16

PART TWO
EXERCISING AND LOVING IT

EXERCISING AND LOVING IT   28
LAWS FOR EXERCISING & LOVING IT   34

PART THREE
PRINCIPLES OF EXERCISE

GETTING STARTED –
GENERAL PRINCIPLES OF EXERCISE   37

PART FOUR
PROGRAMS

APPLYING YOUR LAZY WAY TO ANY ACTIVITY   47
PROGRAMS FOR SUGGESTED ACTIVITIES   53
STEP-UPS & LOVING IT   54
KNEE-UPS & LOVING IT   62
WALKING & LOVING IT   67
WALKING/RUNNING & LOVING IT   70
RUNNING & LOVING IT   73
SWIMMING & LOVING IT   80
STRENGTH TRAINING & LOVING IT   88
STRETCHING & LOVING IT   98

AFTERWORD   103

DEDICATION

To my hero, Hobie Billingsley.
The greatest competitive diving coach in
the history of the sport.

My coach and dear friend

ACKNOWLEDGEMENTS

Harry Mccawley is an associate editor and former sports editor of The Republic newspaper in Columbus, Indiana. His interest, talents, and experience combine to make him the perfect editor for my manuscript. Thanks Harry, for the time, effort, and expertise. I enjoyed our discussions and the editing process, and I learned a lot.

Help is always welcome, and enthusiasm creates miracles. Thanks for the help and enthusiasm from Blake and Lavonne Everroad, Lisa Gundaker, Sherry and Sadie Dettmer, Jim and Carol Blickenstaff, and Nancy and Jim Evans.

Credit is due to Mike McPhearson for an exercise idea which led directly to the Step-Ups and Knee-Up programs.

The editing and input from Ms. Jennifer Underwood Walker are greatly appreciated.

Photography by Jonathon Earley, www.joust.com.

Modeling credits: Neil Bagadiong, Sadie Dettmer, Reginald Jones, Tessa Tucker, Stephen Whited.

PREFACE

This book is based on two discoveries that I learned gradually over a 60-year period of being consistently involved in sports, conditioning, and fitness. In each case these discoveries were "hammered home" by totally unexpected events.

The first discovery was the diagnosis of pre-diabetes by my doctor during a routine physical. So, I wanted and needed to control my blood glucose without medication. I learned immediately that diet alone would not work, and exercise was the only thing left to try.

I also knew that I could not use the high intensity competitive conditioning workouts that I had used all my life. Those workouts would cause me to periodically burn out and quit. My glucose had to be controlled every day. So, I developed the concept I am calling in the first edition, *Your Lazy Way to Great Shape.* And now in the 2nd edition, *The Simple Way to Get Fit* because it works!

The problem with lazy way workouts is that they become boring - precisely because they are easy.

The second discovery occurred while I was doing an easy (and effective) exercise session. It was so easy that I was also watching a video of and old Don Adams sitcom called Get Smart. A running joke in that series involved Adams, as secret agent 86, Maxwell Smart, being sent into harms way. His chief, played by Edward Platt, would tell him something like: "Max, be very careful. You're going to be in the midst of millions of maniacs with machetes who hate men named Max." And Smart would reply, "and loving it."

I was enjoying the comedy segment so much that when I looked at my watch, I found I was 10 minutes over on my exercise time. Without noticing, I'd been exercising too long! At that moment Adams delivered his "and loving it" punch line. The second discovery was hammered home. I realized I was exercising and loving it. That solved the problem of the "too easy, boring" exercise sessions.

So now I have a message: *You can learn to love exercise.* When you do, it will be a part of your lifestyle you will enjoy for the rest of your life.

Then, this confluence of discoveries combined with an even more unexpected event. John Figarelli, the founder and CEO of the National Fitness Museum, nominated me for induction into the National Fitness Hall of Fame.

I was utterly amazed. I simply couldn't imagine that I had accomplished anything that made me worthy of such an honor. Being included with such icons and luminaries as Jack LaLanne, Dr. Kenneth Copper, Arnold Schwarzenegger, and Joseph Pilates was beyond anything I ever imagined.

The National Fitness Hall of Fame gave me both the mandate and responsibility to spread that message. If you take this message to heart, you will *revolutionize your lifestyle with exercise.*

The purpose of this book is to help deliver that messsage.

This book begins with two important sections. Part one is <u>Your Lazy Way to Great Shape</u>. It is essential if you want to love exercise. Part two is <u>Exercising and Loving It</u>. It is essential if you want to be in great shape for the rest of your life.

The third part, <u>Principles of Exercise,</u> gives basic ideas for success in any exercise program.

Part four, <u>Programs,</u> provides detailed plans for applying the lazy way methods to specific activities. I developed these methodologies through direct experiences with each of these activities. I have done and continue to do these programs the way they are described herein. This section also explains how to apply these methods to any activity you like.

PART ONE

YOUR LAZY WAY
TO GREAT SHAPE

YOUR LAZY WAY TO GREAT SHAPE?

Most of us try exercising at one time or another. We join gyms and get pool passes. We buy exercise equipment. We enroll in classes for aerobic dance, Pilates or any other program that might be popular at the time.

Guess what - all these methods work. So, why aren't we all in great shape? For one thing, we're impatient.

When we start, we are hungry for tremendous results ... the sooner the better.

We work hard, too hard. Eventually we burn out. Sound familiar? We have convinced ourselves, through previous attempts, that exercise is much too difficult.

We have developed the attitude that it takes too long, is boring, and can even be expensive. The result of these negative attitudes is that we come to see exercise as unattractive, leading us to exercise improperly.

Inevitably, we quit.

In the end, we lose a critical element in a healthy, happy, successful life - the opportunity to live a lifetime at an optimal fitness level. To have an optimal fitness level, you must exercise successfully. To exercise successfully, you must overcome your negative beliefs. I truly believe that *Your Lazy Way to Great Shape* will help you do just that.

Don't shrug off this concept as something too good to be true. It works. You can get in great shape using a *lazy* approach.

You can find that exercise is easy, not difficult, and doesn't take long. It also doesn't have to be boring or expensive. The lazy way can eliminate your negative attitudes about exercise. Finally, it will be easy for you to reach that optimal fitness level
- great shape.

You can adapt these lazy way methods to any kind of exercise. If you prefer other activities to the programs in this book, that's fine. You can go ahead and renew your gym membership, dust off your old weight bench, oil your exercise bike, or retread you treadmill. Using your lazy way, any form of exercise can be very pleasant and downright fun.

By the way, I am not one of those fitness gurus with big muscles, who devote their entire lives to nothing but exercise. That is fine for those who are so determined but remember - I'm lazy. I prefer to do some basic things consistently. I find this easy and enjoyable and the best approach for realizing most of the appearance benefits that you desire. It is certainly a great way for you to have health and fitness throughout your life.

Quick Start: You probably don't want to read an entire book before getting started. Don't worry. That's perfectly normal. For those who want to get started right away, turn to page 37 and read **How to Do Step-Ups.** Then go to page 39 and start **Your First Session.**

If you don't have an acceptable platform for doing step-ups readily available, try this. Take a slow leisurely walk for 15 consecutive minutes or less depending on how you *feel.* Don't worry about the distance you cover. Then read the rest of the walking program and continue with the walking program as you read this book.

Do read the first three sections as you go! They contain the messages that are critical to your success in any fitness program. The methods, philosophy, and attitudes toward exercise expressed herein are the essential messages.

HEALTH AND FITNESS BENEFITS

Your lazy way to great shape is an easy, efficient way for you to obtain many important health and fitness benefits. These programs offer a number of advantages including:

1. Overcoming obesity.
2. Sustaining weight loss.
3. Cardiorespiratory fitness.
4. Improving your mood and attitude.
5. Increasing energy.

Exercise is critical to overcoming obesity and achieving permanent weight loss for several reasons. It burns calories, increases metabolism, and may aid in reducing caloric intake. Exercise is critical if you want your weight loss to be *fat* loss. If you maintain your current caloric intake and increase your activity level, you *will* lose weight. If you reduce your caloric intake and increase your exercise, you can lose weight quickly.

Cardiorespiratory conditioning is the most important aspect of your physical fitness program. First, exercise provides significant protection for your heart. That's not to say that exercise is a guarantee against heart disease. People in great shape can still have heart attacks. However, this is a very realistic, easy, and effective way to reach a level of fitness to help protect your heart. It could be your most important program for preventing cardiovascular problems.

Taken together, these benefits make you healthier, more productive, and happier. They will make you look and feel better. Your lazy way is virtually essential if you want to have these benefits permanently.

WHY YOUR LAZY WAY TO GREAT SHAPE WORKS

Your lazy way to great shape works by virtue of three principles:
1. Utilization of interval training.
2. Developing an optimal fitness level.
3. Being in great shape.

Interval Training

Years ago, I tried rope skipping to lose and control weight. I also wanted to achieve and maintain cardiorespiratory fitness. I believed a lot of exercise was necessary for weight loss. I also thought I needed to stay in motion for 15 to 20 minutes to expect significant improvements in aerobic fitness.

On my first attempt, I found I could only jump rope continuously for about 90 seconds. It was obvious that if rope jumping were to be an element in my regimen, I had to use a different approach. I decided to adapt a technique called *interval training* to rope skipping.

Interval training was originally developed for highly competitive track and field athletes. Ironically, I first learned of it from Doc Counsilman, the legendary former Indiana University swimming coach. Doc's legend was built on more than his incredible number of national championships, world record holders, and Olympic champions. Key to his phenomenal success was his innovations in sport psychology, biomechanics, and exercise physiology.

Doc was one of the first swimming coaches in the country to introduce interval training to his sport. It became a key component of the Indiana program.

As I considered how effective interval training had been for Doc's swimmers, it occurred to me that it could be modified for personal fitness programs. Instead of making world record holders and Olympic champions out of competitive swimmers, it struck me that this process could also turn unconditioned couch potatoes into physically fit people.

What is Interval Training?

Interval training involves timed rest periods between specific amounts of exercise. Intervals of exercise are followed by intervals of rest. The rest periods might involve standing still and doing nothing; or they might be a continuance of the exercise at reduced intensity. Here's an example of how it might work.

A track and field sprinter might do ten 50-yard dashes at 95% effort in a workout. The athlete would wait two-minute rest intervals between each of the 10 sprints. While the working muscles rest, metabolic wastes are removed from them, and energy sources for the muscles are replenished.

The rest intervals prepare the athlete's muscles for the next sprint, providing greater room for high-intensity training. Interval training was originally designed for high-intensity competitive conditioning workouts. The high intensity of this workout emphasizes speed.

Developing My Jump Rope Program

I wanted to have a high level of cardiorespiratory fitness, but my rope skipping had been too intense, so I needed *lower* intensity. I reasoned that I could lower the intensity of my sessions through interval training.

I knew I could do a few slow continuous steps over the rope easily. With that in mind, I began using low-intensity interval training with my jump rope in a noncompetitive way.

I repeated small numbers of steps between timed rest- intervals in 20-minute sessions. Then, over time, I reduced the interval times and did more continuous steps before each interval.

Eventually I eliminated the intervals, doing 20-minute sessions of continuous slow steps. Then I gradually increased the speed of the steps, thereby increasing the intensity of the sessions. I was doing 2000 steps in 20 minutes within about 60 days. This is still my optimal session for jumping rope.

After experimenting with my number of 20-minute sessions per week, I found that five sessions were effective for losing weight.

I did this without working hard, getting sore, or being the least bit uncomfortable. My excess weight was peeling away. I was in the best aerobic shape of my life, and it was *easy* to do.

It felt so easy I quit calling it a jump rope program and began calling it the *Lope* Rope™ Program. It was a *lazy* way to *great* shape. Also, it was proof that low-intensity interval training was important for personal fitness. Now I believe it is essential for *permanent* fitness.

Optimal Fitness Level

Your Lazy Way to Great Shape allows healthy people to reach their optimal fitness level by exercising for short time periods.

You begin easily with a limited amount of exercise in a set period. For example, my first Lope Rope session was about 300 steps in 20 minutes. I was standing still for most of the 20 minutes.

Then you build an **optimal session** with that desired activity. In subsequent sessions you gradually increase the amount of exercise. More exercise translates into more intensity. When your session is at the right intensity, you can get the results you want. This is your optimal session. My optimal Lope Rope session was 2000 steps in 20 minutes.

Now it's necessary to determine how often to do your optimal session to realize your desired results.

Experiment with the number of times per week you need to get those results. Perform your optimal session with the frequency that provides *the results you want,* and you are at your **optimal performance level**

You might want aerobic fitness, weight loss, strengthening and toning your muscles, or whatever else you choose to pursue. My optimal performance level for the Lope Rope is my optimal session performed every other day.

As you continue with an activity, you can adjust the intensity of the session and your frequency of performing it to perfectly balance your optimal performance level.

If you get *all* the results you want from exercise by doing one activity, your optimal performance level for that activity is also your **optimal fitness level** However, more than one activity might be necessary to provide all the results you want.

Adjusting Your Optimal Fitness Level

Optimal levels for sessions, performance, and fitness vary among individuals for many reasons. Each of us have our individual wants or needs.

Schedules are not always accommodating. Some can manage only a few weekly sessions. So they might need more intensity in their optimal session to have the results they want with less frequent sessions.

Health considerations can either limit the amount of exercise you can do or require that you do more.

Also, you might want more than one cardiorespiratory activity simply for variety (I currently use five activities).

Your optimal fitness level could include any combination of activities. Which activities you choose depends on your specific needs, preferences, and desired results.

Strength training will tend to build strength and muscle mass better than aerobic programs, but aerobic programs will probably do a better job of controlling your cholesterol or lowering your resting pulse rate.

Swimming uses comparatively more upper body muscle mass than walking or running and combining these three activities could give you a more complete fitness program.

And I've found that stretching is the only activity which will keep your joints sufficiently flexible.

So, if you want all these results for your optimal fitness level, you could include all these activities. You could, of course, use other activities to get the same results.

My optimal fitness level changes periodically because I occasionally change my mind about the results I want. Currently, my optimal fitness level includes optimal performance levels with the Lope Rope, knee-ups (defined later), a 35-minute brisk walk, and a combination of walking and jogging. I also do the exercises from my book, *How to Flatten Your Stomach.* I do a strength session with every other flat stomach session.

I vary my routine on alternate days with the Lope Rope and knee-ups. The same holds true for the programs for walking and the combination of walking/jogging. I do the flat stomach exercises nearly every day. When I again change my mind about the results I want, I'll redefine my optimal fitness level.

Effects of Aging on Optimal Levels

As you age, you might need to reduce the exercise in an optimal session. The efficiency of your cardiorespiratory system decreases with age. This decrease is seen in a decreasing maximum achievable heart rate. The decrease in maximum achievable heart rate can be observed from one year to the next. This decrease is slow and gradual, but it is real. Since I first learned of this phenomenon, I have watched my maximum heart rate decrease more than 30 beats per minute for a specific exercise session.

At 69, I am very encouraged - even amazed - that I can still do the optimal jump rope session I developed at age 35. However, if I live long enough the phenomenon of aging will reduce the number of steps I do in 20 minutes. Fewer steps or not, I will: 1) stay just as lazy as I am now, and 2) stay in great shape!

Your lazy way doesn't suddenly end at a given age. My mother passed away just three months short of her 101st year on this planet. During most of her last year, an optimal exercise session for Mom was to get out of bed and move to her chair in the living room. She did this session with the aid of a walker. My sister Jane, a nurse, was our mother's full time care provider. She encouraged this exercise because she could see its positive results.

The results - improved physical, mental and emotional states - were directly observable. Only a few years earlier, Mom was walking a mile a day. The amount of exercise in her session progressively reduced, but she continued to do optimal sessions - the amount of exercise that provided the results she wanted. At age 100, Mom wasn't doing jumping jacks, but she continued to be in great shape!

Speaking of jumping jacks, Jack LaLanne - when I began this writing - was 95 years of age. He still sounded like a young man, had just completed another book, and worked out every day. Jack LaLanne is a fitness legend, and an incredibly inspirational American icon. He maintained an elite level of competitive conditioning from the age of 15. I hoped he would live to 140 just to prove it could be done. And I wanted to be there on that occasion to sing happy birthday - after all, I'd have only been 110.

The world lost the man and gained the legend in 2011.

Be assured that I am not going to do what Jack LaLanne did. I don't believe any other human being has ever done high- intensity competitive conditioning workouts virtually every day of his life for 80 years. I doubt that anyone else ever will.

Hopefully, his commitment to personal fitness will inspire all of us to be in permanent great shape. Compared to what he did, your lazy way provides you with great shape for free.

Maybe you are not sure of the results you want. Well, you are reading this book, so you must want to be in great shape!

Great Shape

"Great shape" describes the combination of all the results you want and need from your exercise program. It is the shape you are in when you reach your optimal fitness level. Most people want results in both their appearance and health.

It is important to define the things you want for yourself. I want my stomach flat, and to be able to see the cuts in my abs (appearance). I want my body weight normal, and my percentage body fat at 15% or less (health and appearance). Since I was diagnosed as pre-diabetic, I want my glucose level under control without insulin or other medicines (health).

There are also physiological markers. My blood pressure should be 120/80 or better, and I want my resting pulse rate at 60 beats per minute or less. Plus, I want my cholesterol and triglycerides at normal levels.

I have designed my optimal fitness level to include optimal performance levels with the Lope Rope, knee-ups, my "flat stomach" exercises, a 35-minute brisk walk, and strength sessions. I'm experimenting with the walking/jogging combo to see if it might help me realize even greater results.

Together, these programs give me all my desired results. The main outcome is that I am in great shape, and I refuse to be anything other than lazy.

Great Shape vs. Competitive Conditioning

I am convinced that a primary reason most people fail to enjoy exercise is because of an attitude that they must *compete* whenever they exercise. They compete against themselves, others, or some imaginary standard they feel must be achieved. This is a reason why they work too hard, burn out, and quit.

Competitive conditioning is intense past the point of pain. You push yourself as hard as you can to do as much as possible. If you are doing less than your opponents, they will have the advantage. Competitive athletes "bust their butts" because they want to win. Doc Counsilman used to describe the phases of his swimmers' workouts as "hurt- pain- agony." It isn't fun.

High intensity competitive conditioning is temporary - considered essential for athletic success but unnecessary afterward. You set goals for each session and each season, with the ultimate goal to be in peak shape at the moment your competition begins.

You are likely to quit your competitive conditioning program when your competition ends. That is because competitive conditioning is *very* hard work. Rational human beings do not generally continue with hard work any longer than necessary.

Further, if you fail to understand that competitive conditioning and optimal fitness are completely different concepts, you tend to think of exercise of any kind as hard work.

So, after your competition is over, you are unlikely to begin exercising in an optimal fitness program. Or, if you do try exercising simply for fitness, you continue to use competitive conditioning. In either case, you will likely quit exercising altogether. Your fitness level will begin to deteriorate, and the deterioration will continue.

Happily, it is very easy to ignore high intensity competitive conditioning workouts and use an optimal fitness program. Why? Competitive conditioning is hard and painful; optimal fitness is easy, fun and fulfilling.

Use a competitive conditioning program if you want to compete. But when your competition days are over, remember an optimal level fitness program called <u>Exercising and Loving It</u>.

PART TWO

EXERCISING AND LOVING IT

EXERCISING and LOVING IT

If you love exercise: 1) it is automatically part of your lifestyle, 2) you are permanently in great shape! Anyone who dreads exercise, regardless of the wonderful results it brings, can simply and easily reverse that feeling and immediately start enjoying these wonderful benefits. This concept combined with your lazy way to great shape guarantees your success!

How Long Does it Take?

Here are three answers:

1. You get results **NOW,** because you start improving with the first movement of your first session. You continue improving with every movement of every session.
2. It takes the rest of your life. That's not a prison sentence. It's common sense - you want to be in great shape for the rest of your life. That can be accomplished easily, comfortably, and pleasantly, if you remain lazy and love it. Emphasize *gradual* and very consistent improvements in your performance. Then just stay with it and you will be in great shape on a permanent basis without ever feeling anything but good!

Oh yeah, I said three answers. What do you imply when you ask the question "How long does it take?"

I suggest the question means you are in a hurry. That question, "How long does it take?" is inappropriate. The third answer to the question is: *do not ask how long it takes!* Be lazy, don't be in a hurry.

The word *workout* is a misnomer applied to personal fitness programs. It was coined to describe competitive conditioning programs. How could you possibly enjoy a **workout?** If it was fun, you would call it play. Your lazy sessions would be better described as *play-outs.*

Avoid pushing yourself too hard. Always do *less* in a session than your capacity. Your optimal performance levels will easily be reached, and you'll **look good and feel great.** The known health benefits are numerous. In fact, you will likely receive even more than we have yet discovered.

The most important reason to use your lazy way is this: *it is easy to be consistent and persistent.* Why? It is an especially pleasant and satisfying method for exercising that provides wonderful results. These are *lifetime* programs you will love.

We all gravitate to what is pleasant and avoid what is not. It's a good bet that if you avoid exercise sessions, you probably find them unpleasant. There are solutions to this problem that will make your sessions pleasant.

Enjoying Your Sessions

<u>Prepare Your Mind</u>

You are subconsciously programmed to think that exercise is too difficult, takes too long, is too boring, and costs money. It's supposed to be intense and competitive. These beliefs tend to emerge when you begin thinking about exercising.

Reject them. Refuse to believe them. Get rid of negative thoughts as soon as they surface. Banish them from your mind. Do not allow them to creep back into your subconscious. Once that's done, reprogram your outlook by preparing for a pleasant experience.

Convincing yourself that exercise is pleasant is simple and easy. Emphasize pleasant thoughts related to your exercise session.

For example, think of walking outside in terms of enjoying a bright, beautiful spring, summer or fall day. Or imagine that your indoor step-ups session is being conducted in a cozy and warm atmosphere on an icy, cold, freezing winter night. Before going to sleep, visualize awakening refreshed, energetic, and ready to take on the world. Then picture yourself starting your day with a pleasant, invigorating exercise session.

Be Comfortable

Comfort is pleasant and a natural partner to lazy. Make your sessions comfortable. You can be comfortable exercising anytime and anywhere.

For instance, you can walk outside even on ridiculously cold and freezing nights and still feel comfortable. When I did that, I would don a snowmobile suit with snowmobile boots and gloves. I also wore a ski mask under the suit's hood. Even in below zero temperatures I didn't experience that first shiver. Nor did I worry about getting mugged by Jack Frost - or for that matter, anyone else. It was far too cold for any self-respecting mugger.

If you have hot sun and a sweltering humid day, a swim is a great way to cool off (the exercise becomes incidental). Use the indoors when you need temperature control (heat or cooling). Use the outdoors when the weather is great.

Always dress appropriately for weather conditions and the intensity you plan to dedicate to your exercise. Remember that raincoats and umbrellas still work just like they always did. Pick your favorite exercise shoe style for comfort.

Focus on Pleasant Activities

You can plan pleasant things to do during an exercise session that will increase the enjoyment of your sessions.

Take a walk and use your cell phone to make a call or text a friend. If you are like a great many of us - and prefer a lazy way of doing things - you will hardly notice you are exercising when you are simply outside, enjoying a beautiful day and talking to a friend on your cell phone.

Plan your sessions to include entertainment you enjoy. And this is *critical,* don't just watch television or listen to music. You don't want some innocuous mediocrity droning in the background. You want to be engrossed in viewing or listening to your *favorite* entertainment. Use music, movies or programs that you love. Download your favorite music and rent your favorite movies and TV programs.

Be entertained while using your lazy way. When you are, your exercise sessions become a time of self-indulgence, absolutely purified because you're not wasting time. You have no need whatever to feel guilty because you are being extremely productive.

Making such activities the *focus* of your session eliminates any negative feelings you might have had about exercise. As you lazily proceed, serendipity occurs.

As you progress using this method, you will find the exercise you are doing enhances the pleasant attitude which you brought into your session. The exercise makes the beautiful day more enjoyable and your conversation more interesting. It makes your music, movie, or program more entertaining. Don't believe me? Try it and you will better understand the meaning of that word serendipity.

Make it Easy

In grade school I noticed a difference between exercise during a training session and exercise in a boxing match, or in a football or basketball game. Even if the intensity levels were the same, workouts were work and playing a game was play. So, exercise could be work or play.

Even when the exercise was intense, at the ripe old age of six or seven it felt more like play than work. It was another interesting principle that I ignored for 50 or 60 years.

So how do you make a training session feel like play? - By applying the Laws for Exercising and Loving It.

LAWS for EXERCISING & LOVING IT

1. *Thou shalt not try hard nor push thyself at all*
2. *Thou shalt not compete against thyself, nor anyone, whilst pursuing thy lazy way*
3. *Thou shalt do less than thou couldst in every exercise session*
4. *Thou shalt not set goals for thy lazy exercise sessions*
5. *Thou shalt not ask, nor even wonder: "How long does it take?"*
6. *Thou shalt be entertained while exercising*
7. *Thou shalt be consistent*
8. *Thou shalt be persistent*
9. *Thou shalt never, never, never quit*
10. *Thou shalt be in great shape*

O.K., I am not Moses. And I must confess, these laws were not handed down from a mountain top. But I swear, they work so well that sometimes it seems like they did come from above.

That sixth law is the key. Include it with the first five and the seventh; eighth, ninth, and tenth laws follow automatically.

Be creative and develop your own ways to make your sessions enjoyable. Remember, positive ... lazy ... comfortable ... pleasant ... easy ... focused on things you enjoy - Exercising and Loving It!

PART THREE

PRINCIPLES OF EXERCISE

GETTING STARTED

See Your Doctor

Get an annual physical exam and talk to your doctor about your exercise program. Get whatever pre-screenings your doctor advises to prevent problems from exercise or to detect any diseases that are still curable. Exercise has a tremendous positive effect on your health, but it is not a guarantee against disease.

The most important consideration for getting started is this: *Always* apply the

<u>LAWS of EXERCISING and LOVING IT</u>

GENERAL PRINCIPLES OF EXERCISE

Frequency

To consistently move toward an optimal session, you should exercise at least three times a week. You can exercise as often as every day but don't push yourself or try hard. You should feel refreshed at the end of each session. If you are less than refreshed at the end of a session, either decrease the exercise in a session for a while or give yourself more time between exercise periods. Be lazy.

You may be able to continue doing an optimal session by exercising only twice a week or even less. This is another reason why it is easy to be consistent and persistent with these programs. However, you may need more to realize all the *results* you want. So, your optimal performance and/or your optimal fitness level may require more than two sessions per week.

Your optimal performance level may be found at **any** level of a program depending on how you adapt to it. Experiment with the number of times per week to do your optimal sessions. Make them provide what you want from the exercise. Adjust your frequency for performing them to get your optimal fitness level.

Be Consistent and Persistent!

It will probably take you some significant time to reach an optimal performance level. That's good! Take as long as necessary. If it takes a year or longer, who cares? Whether you exercise or not, that time is going to pass. You can do nothing for a year and just be a year older. Or you can be a year older, *feel* a year younger, and be in the best shape of your life!

Be consistent. Do at least two, and preferably three sessions each week You should also be persistent. If you miss an exercise period because of a holiday, get back in the routine. If you miss a week or two because of an illness or injury, you return when you can. You might miss a month or longer because of some major lifestyle change. Get restarted!

Even after you get into great shape, you might take time off. It's not a crime. For whatever reason, whatever length of time, if you are interrupted, you can always come back to your program. Interruptions don't have to be endings. They do not mean you have *quit.* Your program doesn't end unless you quit.

Don't ever quit! Be consistent and persistent. You will be in great shape for the rest of your life, which will likely be significantly longer, healthier, more productive, and happier.

Pulse rate vs. Performance

Your Lazy Way to Great Shape emphasizes the amount of exercise in your sessions rather than your target heart rate. This makes it simpler and easier for you to develop an optimal session. However, it might be interesting to monitor your pulse rate as you move toward that optimal session.

Depending on the exercise, you can monitor your pulse rate at any stop in your session or immediately after it. To check your pulse, place the first finger of one hand against the pulse on the wrist of the opposite hand. Count the pulse beats for six seconds and place a zero after the number of beats (example: if you count 10 beats, place a zero after the 10, for approximately 100 beats per minute).

It's a good idea to use a timer in counting to six seconds since few of us can estimate time accurately.

Coaching tip 1: Pulse rate monitors are available in sporting goods stores. They are not necessary for your success, but you may find them interesting and worth using. **Caution:** Don't become reliant on a pulse rate monitor. If you are using one and it breaks, or you lose it, or don't have it with you, or you don't want to bother with it, etc. - well, you get the picture. Just keep exercising and don't sweat the small stuff.

Reverse-goal: At first, keep your pulse rate *less* than 120 beats/minute during your early sessions. A higher pulse rate is likely to cause you to wear out and quit before you've completed your exercise. As your fitness level improves (it will - **dramatically),** you will be able to reach and maintain your **target** heart rate easily for the whole session.

Don't worry about your target heart rate. When you think you've reached an optimal performance session, you will likely find that you are within your target heart rate parameters. If not, you can modify your sessions to adjust your heart rate.

To determine target heart rate for an aerobic exercise session:

1. Subtract your age from 220. This is your projected maximum heart rate.
2. Multiply your projected maximum heart rate by 85%, and then multiply it by 70%.
3. The results of step two are the high and low limits for your target heart rate in **beats/minute.**
4. Your average **heart** rate should be about 75-80% of your projected maximum heart rate.

Important: The above formula is generally used for determining pulse rate parameters for aerobic fitness. *Lower* pulse rates are *more* appropriate for many results. For example, my pulse rate while walking is never over 67% and averages about 60%. However, a 35-minute brisk walk consistently drops my blood glucose from a high spike to a normal range. My pulse rate averages about 75-80% during an optimal Lope

Rope session. But the Lope Rope is *less* efficient than walking for controlling my glucose level.

Disclaimer: My statements about controlling blood glucose are based on my own monitoring of my blood glucose. While they have been true for me for more than three years of monitoring, they cannot be generalized to others. I am not prescribing any method or technique for the controlling of blood glucose for diabetics. I mean only to illustrate the principle that lower pulse rate exercise is worthwhile. I especially like this illustration because it came as a complete surprise to me.

Using Logs

Logs are extremely valuable with these programs. They serve as proof that you are getting into great shape. If you are not working hard, there's a tendency to feel your sessions are getting you nowhere. Your logs will refute that "feeling" with documentary evidence that you are getting into great shape even though you feel lazy.

Record every session and be sure the records are easy to read. I usually prefer paper log sheets to using a computer. I keep mine on top of my main desk in full view all the time. Samples of what to include in your log are included in the sections for each program.

Design these log sheets to show as many sessions in a single glance as possible. I have 12 weeks on one side of an 8½" x 11" sheet of paper. This makes it easy to see my improvement over the course of months or even years.

After you have been with a program for a while, you will be amazed at how much your performance has improved - even though you have been lazy. Since it has been so easy to improve so much, you will have visual proof to encourage you to keep moving toward your optimal performance level. And, it has been so easy to get to that point that it will be easy to stay there. You simply, and lazily, are in great shape.

If you would prefer not to make your own log sheets, you can order paper log sheets for your program from https://ExercisingAndLovingIt.com. If you do order log sheets, don't wait until you get the sheets to begin. You can copy the data from your first sessions into new log sheets when you receive them. Start **NOW!**

Cool-down and Stretching

After your sessions, be sure to cool down by taking leisurely walks. Cool down for at least five minutes after your exercise until your pulse rate is 100 beats/minute or less. Several minutes of stretching will help you to cool further. Stretching can be part of your cooling down period.

Stretching will keep your joints and muscles flexible and supple. Cooling down and stretching helps you to avoid soreness and injuries. Both will help you feel good after your sessions and make it easier to stay consistent and persistent.

Coaching tip 2: You do need a watch or clock with a second hand or numeric display of seconds. You must be able to see it easily while exercising.

Coaching tip 3: Use **LAW 6.** First decide what you want to use for *entertainment.* Then get it ready to use, then start exercising and loving it!

PART FOUR

PROGRAMS

APPLYING YOUR LAZY WAY
to ANY ACTIVITY

First you must decide what you want to do. This book includes prepared programs for step-ups, knee-ups, walking, a combined walking and jogging program, running, swimming, stretch cords, and stretching. If you prefer any of these activities, you can turn straight to that program.

All the above programs were created using the methods listed below. You can use the methods to develop your programs for exercise bikes, treadmills, ellipticals, rowing machines, roller skates or bicycles. They could also be critical factors for cross country skiing, pole walking or *any other exercise activity.*

These methods are vital for having permanent optimal performance levels.

If you like aerobic dance, kung fu fighting, all-around gymnastics, pole-vaulting, or any other appropriate physical activity, go for it. Any activity you enjoy is a good activity for your personal fitness program.

Use the different ideas for enjoying sessions from each of the different activities' sections. Also, be creative and explore your own ideas for making your sessions pleasant.

Log the pertinent information from every session immediately. The activity and the principles you use to create your sessions determine what comprises pertinent information.

Any of the methods listed below might be exactly right for the activity you want to use. Or you can use any combination of these methods to create a perfectly lazy way. Also, you might find or invent other methods you personally prefer. Nobody knows your preferences better than you. Design programs the way you want, and you will never, never, never want to quit.

Enjoy your lazy sessions and be at optimal fitness level - great shape- permanently- and loving it!

Short Single Intervals

1. Begin with a single interval of slow and easy, but continuous movements of an activity. The session should consist of one untimed, unmeasured session. Move for small amounts of either time or distance. Examples: a bicycle ride of fifteen, ten or five minutes ... maybe even *less,* or a walk to the end of the street and back, or around the block, or maybe a little farther.

2. Gradually increase your continuous movement. To do this it's best to maintain your pace and increase your time or distance. Do this lazily.

3. When either your time or distance is sufficient for your session, you can adjust the intensity of the movement. Do so by increasing your pace for the movement. Do this gradually and lazily.

4. With experience, you will create a balance between your pace and your time or distance that provides your optimal session.

5. Experiment with the number of optimal sessions per week necessary to have your optimal performance

level for the activity. This method is illustrated in the Walking program.

Idle Rest Intervals

Define a session by either its length of time or distance. For instance, a Step-Ups session is defined as 20 minutes (time) without considering the number of steps. By contrast the Swimming Program defines a session according to distance (800 yards) without regard to time.

1. Always begin with short, easy, and *untimed* exercise intervals of the activity.

2. Follow each exercise interval with long, idle, and untimed rest intervals. All your rest intervals must provide enough time to fully recuperate before the next exercise interval.

3. Repeat unplanned numbers of exercise and rest intervals for the duration of your session. Duration means either time or distance.

4. Decide the duration of your session using a: or b:

   a. Time: How many minutes in your session?

   b. Distance: How far will you go? Your first sessions should be of a shorter distance than you ultimately want for the session. For example, begin your swimming sessions at 400 yards and later increase it to 800 yards.

5. The durations of exercise intervals are based entirely on how you feel. *Feel lazy!*

6. In subsequent sessions, make gradual increases in each untimed exercise interval.

7. Begin timing your rest intervals. You should still be doing short, easy exercise intervals. Feel comfortable and continue to feel lazy as you begin to use timed rest- intervals.

8. Use the same time for each rest interval.

9. Continue increasing your exercise intervals while gradually decreasing your timed rest intervals. *Be lazy* as you do so.

10. Gradually and lazily increase the exercise intervals and decrease the rest interval time until the rest intervals are eliminated. Do this over an unplanned number of sessions.

Now you are doing the activity continuously for the full planned duration. Or you might find an optimal session *before* the rest intervals are eliminated.

Neither the total amount of exercise in a timed session, nor the total amount of time in a distance session is pre- determined.

Optimizing Idle Rest Intervals

When you are moving continuously for the entire session, it's important to find an optimal session for the activity. Here's how:

1. If your session is based on a given length of time, it's okay to increase the pace during the allotted time to find your optimal session.

2. If your session is based on distance, you can reduce the time for completing the prescribed distance.
3. After finding an optimal session, experiment with the number of times per week necessary to have your optimal performance level for the activity.

Avoid trying hard or pushing yourself at all.

Low and High Intensity Intervals

You can see this method in the Knee-ups program. It's also in the combination Walking/Running program. The Walking/Running program begins with long, low intensity sessions. As intensity increases, the length of the sessions shortens.

The Knee-ups program is based on 20-minute sessions consisting of 10 two-minute sets. Each set consists of a lower intensity step-ups interval and a higher intensity knee-ups interval.

1. Develop an optimal session in a lower intensity activity, e.g., walking.

2. Alternate long intervals of the lower intensity activity with short intervals of a higher intensity activity, e.g., running.You are substituting the lower intensity activity for idle rest intervals.

3. Gradually increase the higher intensity intervals and decrease the lower intensity intervals. You can continue until the lower intensity intervals are ended. Or you might find an optimal session before the lower intensity intervals are eliminated. Don't forget to be lazy.

4. If you eliminate the lower intensity intervals and still need more exercise, gradually increase the exercise for the higher intensity activity until you find an optimal session.

5. Experiment with the number of times per week necessary to have your optimal performance level for the activity.

Perceived Exertion

This method is illustrated by the Strength and Stretching programs. It operates well when a session is defined by neither time nor distance. In both of these programs a session is defined by the amount of exercise performed, e.g., number of exercises and number of repetitions.

1. Exercise till you *feel* you have reached 75-80% of your potential to continue. Use subjective perception to determine when you reach 75-80%. Be lazy with your subjective perception.

2. Relax at idle till you are completely refreshed.

3. Repeat steps 1 and 2 until you feel the session is complete.

4. As your sessions become easier, you will probably increase the amount of exercise in them. However, even after increasing the exercise, it should never feel more strenuous to do a session. This is because you continue to use the same perception of your exertion- 75 to 80%.

The length of your rest intervals is always determined by perception. Simply wait until you are ready to continue.

PROGRAMS for SUGGESTED ACTIVITIES

Stretching must be included as a part of any program. Also, a cardiorespiratory program is advisable for receiving the health benefits of a personal fitness program. Finally, strength training may not be necessary, but it is extremely worthwhile. Including strength training provides you with a complete fitness program. So, start with a cardiorespiratory program accompanied with proper stretching. Add strength training later as your fitness improves.

The cardiorespiratory programs discussed in this book are step-ups, knee-ups, walking, a combined walking and jogging program, running, and swimming Deciding which cardiorespiratory program to use first could be based on necessity and/or convenience. You might want to swim, but the closest swimming area is two hours away. Or, you might want to walk, but you are surrounded by busy streets with no sidewalks. If such problems stop you from using the programs discussed herein, buy a treadmill, jump rope, or whatever else suits your wants and needs. Perhaps you already own a good rowing machine, elliptical, exercise bike, or some other equipment. Great! Simply apply the lazy way methods to create your program for that activity.

If you are not sure what you prefer, start with
STEP-UPS YOUR LAZY WAY.

STEP-UPS & LOVING IT

Step-ups provide a wonderful opportunity for pleasant exercising. You can do them anywhere - outside in nice weather or inside when there is ice on the deck. You can do them next to the bed immediately after awakening in the morning (an excellent choice) or you can watch a favorite TV program in the living room while you are exercising.

My favorite time is while I am listening to an oldies radio station. I look forward to the sessions because the exercise makes me more alert and being more alert *enhances the pleasure of listening to the music.*

How to Do Step-Ups

This program is characterized by ease and simplicity. The activity is to repeat stepping up onto a platform then back down again. The platform can be as simple as a stair step. You put one foot on top of your platform, then the other foot. Then step back down with your first foot, followed by stepping down with your second foot.

So, the movement has four parts: 1) forward and up with one foot, 2) forward and up with the other foot, 3) back and down with the first foot, 4) back and down with the second foot. Count the completion of all four parts as one repetition.

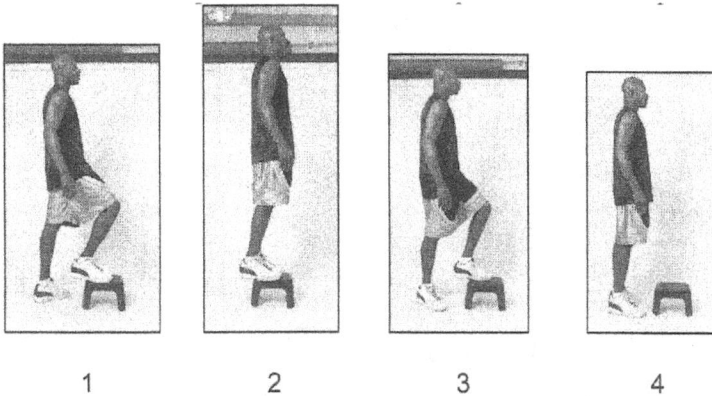

| 1 | 2 | 3 | 4 |

These steps are easy to do unless your step is too high, so be sure your step is low enough to be in your comfort zone. You should get into a consistent cadence in a session, and you can do that with a rhythmic counting of your steps.

This program is based on 20-minute sessions. Your optimal session will be the number of steps in 20 minutes that provide the results you want.

You set your own rules. If your session becomes continuous at a quick pace for 20 minutes and you still want more exercise, increase the height of your step. Or, if 20 minutes with sets of few steps between intervals at a *slow* pace is too laborious, you can switch to a lower step.

This program is simple and convenient enough to do every day. I suggest three to five sessions per week for your optimal performance level.

What You Need

If you have a stepstool or a staircase in your home, you have everything you need for **STEP-UPS** &

LOVING IT. If not, you can buy an inexpensive stepstool at most discount department stores. If you are using your staircase, be sure to use the *bottom* step.

If you're a do-it-yourself type and want to improvise a platform for step-ups, be sure it is sturdy. Also, be aware of the potential for slippage. Make sure the bottom doesn't slip across the floor and your feet don't slip on its surface.

Coaching tip 4: If you want to make your own inexpensive step-up system, begin with a 2" x 10" board. Cut four sections, each 15" long. One section, lying flat, is 1¾" in height; a stack of two is 3½ inches. A stack of three is 5¼", and a stack of four is seven inches. Seven inches is comparable to the height of many stepstools, and the bottom stair that I use is 7½ inches. A couple of well-placed nails or wood screws between any set of two pieces will keep them from slipping.

There are two distinct advantages to this system. It makes it easy to adjust the height of your step to best facilitate your step- ups. Later, you can also adjust the height to best perfect your optimal performance level.

The important thing to keep in mind is that nothing *is more important than to start exercising right now. Don't be delayed by the process of developing a perfect system.* Unless you have the necessary tools and materials at hand to build it now, use a stepstool or stair.

Your First Session

For your first session, try five repetitions lifting one foot up first and then do five reps lifting the other foot first. Remember your lazy laws. Don't try too hard or push yourself. Above all, avoid any tendency to compete against yourself. If five repetitions are anything other than lazy, do fewer. A given number of repetitions with one foot first, followed by the same number of repetitions with the other foot first complete one **exercise interval.**

Example: five repetitions leading with the left foot, followed immediately by five repetitions leading with the right foot equal one exercise interval of ten reps.

After your **first** exercise interval, rest if you need to feel completely recuperated and be sure that you are ready to go on to a second exercise interval.

This recuperation period is your **rest interval.** In the beginning, do *not* time either your rest or exercise intervals. Simply pay attention to how you feel. The combination of an exercise interval and a rest interval is one **set.**

After your first rest interval, do a second set with the same number of repetitions as your first set. Repeat doing sets with the same number of reps and with untimed rest intervals for 20 minutes.

If your 20 minutes ends in the middle of an exercise interval, stop. Count the number of sets you complete in

20 minutes. Add any reps from an unfinished interval to your total.

In your first session, you should be standing still and doing nothing for most of the 20 minutes. Always leave something in reserve. Do *less* **than you could do in every session!** Be lazy.

Logging Step-Ups & Loving It

Be sure to record every session on your log sheet as per this sample log sheet entry. Include the categories from this sample on your log sheet. Place the number of

Date	Sets	Rest Interval	Reps/Set	+	Total Reps
05/01	9	untimed	10	3	93

completed sets under the heading **Sets** on your sheet. Place any repetitions from an unfinished exercise interval under the + column. Multiply the number of sets by the number of reps per set, then add any reps from the + column for your total number of reps.

This sample log shows a first session on May 1. The rest- intervals were untimed. Nine complete sets with 10 reps were performed. In each exercise interval, five reps lifting one foot up first was followed by five reps with the other foot up first (10 reps/set). The total reps were 93 (nine sets x 10 reps per set + three reps).

Your Optimal Performance Level

You might find it easy to add a repetition or two to your sets in the next session. Or you might reduce a repetition or two from your sets. Stay lazy. Whether or not you add, subtract, or keep your repetitions the same, keep your intervals untimed. Mark your log sheet immediately after each session so you can monitor your activity. As you continue, you will see gradual increases in both your number of sets and your total number of repetitions.

In subsequent sessions, add repetitions to your sets until you are doing 20 reps/set (10 reps lifting one foot up first, then 10 with the other foot first). After doing your first session with 20-rep exercise intervals, determine the length of your first rest-interval.

Establish the length of your first rest-interval by timing how long it takes to feel completely recuperated and ready to start the second set. Then use that time for all your rest intervals in the session.

Example: You find that 60 seconds is enough time to completely recuperate. So, you use 60 seconds for all the rest-intervals in your session.

Your exercise intervals remain untimed.

When you want more exercise, your best strategy is to reduce your rest interval time. If your first timed rest interval was 60 seconds, try dropping each interval in a session to 55 seconds. Don't push and avoid reducing interval times too much or too soon. Stay with a given rest interval until you *know* it will be easy to lower it. Drop five seonds at a time if that works well for you. Drop less interval time if that works better. Be lazy.

When you reduce your rest interval time to 30 seconds, try combining sets and increasing intervals. Example: You are doing 20-rep sets with 30-second rest intervals. Now, you begin doing 40-rep sets with 60-second rest intervals. Then you again reduce interval times gradually over an unplanned number of sessions to 30 seconds. Stay lazy.

Now you can combine 40-rep sets to make sets of 80 reps while increasing your rest interval time. Since you have doubled your reps/set, you might want to try a longer interval. Instead of using 60 seconds, try increasing the rest interval to 90 seconds, or two minutes or longer. Then repeat reducing intervals down to 30 seconds as you did before. Do this again with 160 reps.

You will likely be able to combine two sets of 160 reps for a set of 320 reps. However, you may not have enough time to do two sets of 320 reps with a rest interval. If not, you do the first set of 320, use a new interval, and then finish your 20-minute session with continuous step-ups.

Now, using the same technique as before, move your interval time down in five second reductions. As you reduce the rest interval times, add steps to the end of your second set Adding steps will keep your session 20 minutes long. Ultimately, you might eliminate the rest intervals and do one continuous set lasting the whole 20 minutes.

A continuous 20 minutes of any specific number may be your optimal session. Try the number of step-ups/sessions you are doing for the number of days/week that you want to do them. If you are getting the results you want, you are at optimal performance level. If not, you might want to increase the height of your step and/or speed up your pace.

Adjust your pace and/or height of your step until you are getting the results you want. Make these adjustments lazily.

Important: You might find your optimal session anywhere from your first session to any session described above. A session that provides the results *you* want, when performed your given number of times per week, is exactly right for you - your optimal performance level for **STEP-UPS** & **LOVING IT.**

<u>Coaching</u> <u>tip 5:</u> If your optimal session is a continuous 20-minute session, you might want to invest in an inexpensive metronome to make your sessions more pleasant. It allows you to quit counting your steps and simply match the movement of your feet to the metronome's cadence. Now you can quit counting while you think about other things, listen to music, watch television, converse, talk on your cell phone, etc. Does the idea of *play-outs* make more sense now?

Also, <u>www.metronomeonline.com</u> lets you use your computer as a metronome for free. It is easy to use. And there are free apps for mobile phones.

Set the metronome for the same cadence as the number of times you move your feet in one minute. One rep is four movements (up, up, down, down= four), so multiply the number of reps you do in one minute by four. Example: four movements/rep x 30 reps/minute= 120 movements/minute. So, if you do 30 reps/minute (120 movements/minute), you set the metronome at 120 *beats/minute.*

Stretching for Step-Ups/Knee-Ups & Loving It

Do stretching exercises one, two, three, and four from **STRETCHING** & **LOVING** IT during the cooling down period after each session.

KNEE-UPS & LOVING IT

Adding "knee-ups" to your step-ups is a great way to enhance your program. The knee-up movement increases the range of motion for your legs and makes them more fit. Your muscles will get more strength and endurance throughout their whole range of motion, and your ankle, knee, and hip joints will gain more flexibility. These advantages can make dramatic improvements in the appearance of your legs.

The knee-up is a more dynamic movement than the step-up. As a result, it increases the intensity of your exercise. This raises your average heart rate during a session causing an increase in cardiorespiratory fitness with all the corresponding benefits.

Important: The knee-up movement can be very good for some *lower back problems.*

So, if you want more of these results, knee-ups are a fun, easy, lazy way to get them.

Guiltless Loafing - Your Lazy Way to Great Shape

I absolutely love this program. I do it while watching different short comedies on video disc. I enjoy these comedies so much that I can't wait to watch them. Since I only indulge myself in this entertainment while exercising, I can't wait to exercise.

I become much more focused on the humor than on the exercise. Except for the monotonous metronome droning in the background, I would forget that I am exercising at all.

If I were lounging on the couch in the middle of the afternoon watching slapstick humor and dumb jokes (the Three Stooges, Get Smart, Married with Children, etc.), be assured that I would be severely criticized for loafing.

In 'fact, I would feel terrible guilt, bordering on worthlessness, for loafing.

During these sessions, I feel like I'm loafing even though I know I'm being extremely productive and even *look* like I'm working.

Knee-ups are the perfect disguise for a pleasant interlude of guiltless loafing - like the subtitle says - "your lazy way to great shape!"

How to Do Knee-ups

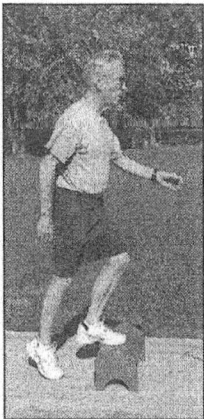 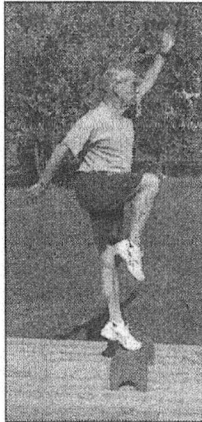 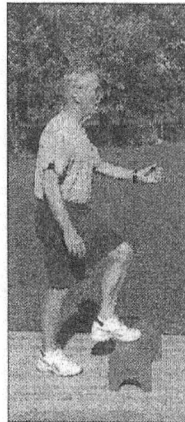 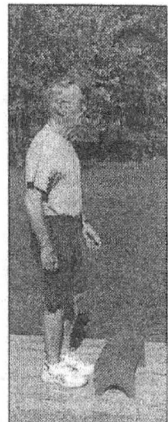

Picture 1   Picture 2   Picture 3   Picture 4

As with step-ups, four parts of the movement equal one repetition of the exercise. The first part is exactly the same as step-ups. Lift one foot and place it on the platform (picture 1).

Then lift the other foot and continue lifting, driving the knee forcefully up as close to your chest as possible. Allow your knee to bend as it moves upward. At the peak height of your knee, it should be bent so your heel is close to your rear (picture 2).

While your knee is moving upward, swing your opposite arm forward and up to be on balance during the movement. As you drive the knee up, you also raise the heel of your first foot as high as you can. At the peak of the knee-up, all your weight will be supported on the ball of your lead foot (also picture 2).

Lower your second foot back to starting position, keeping the lead foot on the platform (picture 3).

Now lower your lead foot back to starting position for one rep (picture 4).

Lead your next rep with the other foot, driving the opposite knee up, swinging the opposite arm forward and raising the heel of your support foot as high as you can.

From Step-Ups to Your Knee-Ups Program

The Knee-Ups program is a continuation of the 20-minute per session Step-Ups program. Much of it remains the same. Follow the same methods to enjoy the exercise. Use the same platform, and the same places for doing your sessions.

Also, the stretching and cool-down is the same as for your Step-Ups sessions and, if you like using a metronome for Step- Ups, continue using it for this program. Just continue with the same cadence.

Your First Knee-Ups Session

Before beginning your Knee-Ups program, you should be doing 20 minutes of continuous step-ups without rest intervals. If you are, it will be easy to gradually add knee-ups to your sessions. If you aren't, the increased intensity will be too great.

Divide the number of steps you are doing by 10 to get the number to do in each two-minute set. Then continue doing the same number of steps in each two-minute set replacing some step-ups with knee-ups.

Now divide each of your 10 two-minute sets into an interval for regular step-ups plus a second interval for knee-ups.

Do the same number of reps you used in the regular step-ups program. But now begin replacing some of the regular step-ups with knee-ups. Example: If you're doing 600 step-ups in 20 minutes, that equates to 60 steps in each two minutes. For your first Knee-Ups session, try 56 step-ups in the first interval and four knee-ups in the second interval of each of your ten sets.

Date	Sets	Intervals SU + KU	Total steps
07/25	10 x 2 mins	56 + 4	600

You will need a different log sheet for knee-ups. Log the above example using this sample log as shown. The log shows 600 total steps in a 20-minute session. The total steps are 10 sets x 56 step-ups/set= 560 step-ups+ 10 sets x 4 knee-ups/set= 40 knee-ups. 560 total step-ups+ 40 knee-ups= 600 total steps.

Six hundred steps in 20 minutes are not a rule or even a recommendation. You might want to do more or less. The idea is to determine the intensity of your sessions based on the results you get from them.

To increase your number of knee-ups, gradually replace step-ups with knee-ups in each set. It is easiest to replace them one per set at a time. Increase more per set if you like but keep the Laws for Exercising & Loving It firmly in mind.

Your Optimal Performance Level

As you add knee-ups, your sessions will become more intense. The more intense they become, the more gradually you should add knee-ups. You can change one set per session.

Example: Change your first set to 55 step-ups+ 5 knee- ups; and stay with 56 + 4 for your 2nd through 10th sets. Next session: 1st **two** sets, 55 step-ups + 5 knee-ups; **third** through 10th sets 56 + 4, etc. This is very gradual and extremely effective. *Your current session never feels harder than the previous one.* So, you can increase your intensity as much as you want; and you *can* stay lazy and be in great shape!

I have continued this method for several years. I am currently doing intervals of 7 step-ups and 59 knee-ups. I like to do 66 steps per set on a 7 1/2" high platform. My pulse rate averages just over 70% of my projected maximum heart rate.

As I can do so easily, I plan to continue gradually replacing step-ups with knee-ups to see if knee-ups will provide a heart rate of 80%. This is not a goal, but only to satisfy my curiosity.

I refuse to break any of the Laws for Exercising & Loving It to increase the intensity. So, if my heart rate never reaches 80%, my curiosity will be satisfied, and I will continue at a lazy intensity.

You can continue replacing step-ups until you reach a continuous 20-minute session of only knee-ups. But you will probably get the results you want by doing much less. Be lazy.

When you find your optimal session, experiment with the number of sessions per week you need for your optimal performance level. Mine is every other day. Sometimes I wish it was more often.

WALKING & LOVING IT

You will find this program simple to follow, satisfying, and easy to do. It involves gradual increases in session time and does not employ rest intervals. You can add to the pleasure by bringing along a portable system for playing your favorite music.

Begin with a slow leisurely walk. Don't worry about the distance. Dedicate 15 minutes or less depending on how *you feel.* Be aware of how you feel before, during, and after the walk. If you begin to tire, slow down or stop. Do less than you know you can do. If you feel better at the end than you did at the beginning, you are setting an excellent pace.

Use the way you feel to decide when to add time to your walk. If you are refreshed at the end of your first walk, increase your time in your next session. Increase your time by five minutes or less. If your first walk was anything less than lazy and you feel fatigued, walk fewer minutes next time.

Walk at least every other day or as often as five days a week. So long as you feel good after your walk, you can increase your time in the next session. Do this lazily. Always use five minutes or *less* for your increased times.

Eventually, you might find it easy to walk for a full hour. This is not a goal, and you should not set a goal. You might find your optimal walking session in less than one hour (mine is 35 minutes). Remember that your optimal session is defined by the results you want. Don't worry about how long it takes you to develop an optimal walking session. Keep in mind that the results will be the same regardless of how long it takes to have an optimal session. Always pay attention to how you feel. *Avoid pushing yourself* and *enjoy your walks.*

Maintaining a leisurely pace for an hour may provide your optimal walking session. If you need more exercise, increase your pace until you have an optimal walking session. A nonstop walk of one-hour or *less,* and/or a distance of 3½ miles or less should provide you with an optimal session.

Reverse-goal: walk no more than one hour, and 3½ miles or less in each walking session.

For your optimal performance level, three days per week may be enough, or you might want four or five sessions. The key is to get the results you want from walking. Experiment with the number of optimal session walks you do per week. Five sessions per week could provide an optimal performance level for walking, but not an optimal, fitness level. If so, keep walking and try adding **SWIMMING & LOVING IT** or **WALKING/RUNNING & LOVING IT.** Or, if you like jumping rope, see the Lope Rope Program at www.loperope.com.

The more intense programs will improve your cardiorespiratory fitness. When you are using another optimal performance program, try alternating it with your Walking Program. There is no reason ever to work hard to be at your optimal fitness level.

Stretching & Logging for Walking & Loving It

Do stretching exercises one, two, three, and four from **STRETCHING** & **LOVING** IT during the cooling down period after each session.

Use a log sheet to keep track of your sessions. This will help you to be consistent and persistent with your program. Your log sheet will prove you are getting into great shape, even though you are being lazy. In keeping your log, remember that we are doing this the lazy way. There is not that much information to record for a walking program. The date and number of minutes walking may be all you need. Nonetheless, it is **important** that you maintain your logs. It is essential for seeing the results you get from using your lazy way.

Use the example to design your log sheet. The example illustrates a

Date	Minutes	Distance
9/23	15	unmeasured

walking session on September 23 of 15 minutes duration, with the distance unmeasured.

Coaching tip 6: It isn't necessary to consider the distance you walk in your optimal walking session. However, if you want to know the distance you are walking, inexpensive pedometers ($10.00 or less) will measure the distance you walk within acceptable accuracy. A pedometer is certainly not necessary for your success in a walking program. I don't use one, but if they make any aspect of your exercise easier, I'm all for it. Easier is lazier, and I'm lazy, remember? If interested, enter pedometers into a computer's search engine, or check a local sporting goods store. Smart phones also have a "health" app you can download.

WALKING/RUNNING & LOVING IT

Develop an optimal performance level walking program before beginning this program. Walking will build physiological foundations that will make it much safer and easier to run. These foundations include strengthening your muscles and joints as well as, cardiorespiratory improvements. Your optimal performance level walking program will make running safer.

As with your walking program, you can use any portable system for your favorite music. Use music or some other favorite diversion to make your walking/running sessions more pleasant. This is essential to effect a change in your lifestyle! The advantages of adding running to your walking are: 1) since running requires more energy than walking, you can burn a given number of calories in less time, 2) because running requires more oxygen consumption per minute than walking, it offers more cardiorespiratory fitness, 3) running requires more strength than walking ... resulting in the improvement in the strength, tone, and shape (appearance) of the muscles of your legs.

Start each session of your walking/running program by walking. Don't worry about your speed or distance. Lazy, slow, and short distance is the right approach. You should alternate walking and running for the number of minutes on the chart according to the session you are using. Session A consists of 8½ minute sets repeated 7 times. Each set is an eight-minute walking interval followed by a 30 second running interval.

Session	Time/Set	# Sets	Time Time Walking+Running	Total Walk	Total Run	Total Session
A	8½ min	7	8 m + 30 s	56 m	3½min	59½min
B	8 min	7	7½ m + 30 s	52½ m	3½min	56 min
C	8 min	7	7m + 1 m	49 min	7min	56 min
D	7½ min	7	6½m + 1 m	45½ m	7 min	52½ min
E	7 min	7	6m + 1 m	42 m	7 min	49 min
F	6½ min	7	5½m + 1 m	38½ m	7min	45½ min
G	7 min	6	5½m + 1½ m	33 m	9 min	42 min
H	6½ min	6	5m +1½ m	30 min	9 min	39 min
I	6 min	6	4½m + 1½ m	27 min	9 min	36min
J	6½ min	5	4½m +2 m	22½min	10 min	32½min

K	6 min	5	4m +2 m	20 min	10 min	30 min

Session A provides 56 minutes of walking time, 3½ minutes of running time, for a total session time of 59½ minutes.

If you are doing a 60-minute optimal walking session, this first step will be very easy for you. If you have not developed an optimal walking session, this step could be much too difficult. If your optimal walking session is less than one hour, I would *not* suggest running.

To increase your running, move from less intense sessions (A) toward more intense sessions (K). Change sessions only when you can do your current step lazily.

Avoid pushing yourself and *take all the time you need.* Don't consider the distance covered during your sessions.

Session A might be your optimal session. If not, move down the sequence of sessions on the chart till you have found an optimal session.

Important: Any session on the chart, A - K might serve as your optimal session. Your optimal session is the amount of exercise in a specific time period that can provide the results *you* want. Find an optimal session that feels lazy.

When you have found an optimal session, experiment with the number of sessions per week you feel are necessary for an optimal performance level. After you find the frequency for performing your sessions that produces the results desired, you have an optimal performance level for **Walking/Running** & **Loving** It.

Stretching for Walking/Running & **Loving** It

When you finish a session, you should stay on your feet and continue to move around at a leisurely pace. Stretch at the ankles, knees, and hips to avoid stiffness. Do stretching exercises one, two, three, and four from **STRETCHING** & **LOVING IT** during the cooling down period after each session. Cooling down and stretching should last for at least five minutes.

Log every session. It allows you to see the progress you have made to great shape. Your log should include all the information you see on the sample log. The sample shows session H being performed on August 26. Each set was 6½ minutes. The lazy exerciser did six sets of five-minute walks + 1½-minute runs. This provided 30 minutes of walking, nine minutes of running, and a total 39 minutes of exercising.

Date	Time/Set	#Sets	Time Time Walking+Running	Walk	Run	Session
08/26	6½min	6	5m+1½m	30min	9 min	39min

RUNNING & LOVING IT

<u>Coaching tip 7:</u> If you want to run, start with **WALKING YOUR LAZY wAY** and put on hold that plan to win the Boston Marathon. At least be lazy enough to delay running until you are doing an optimal walking session (lazily).

A continuous running session of 20 minutes is the most intense exercise session in this book It is not necessary for an optimal fitness level. However, running might meet your personal desires and preferences for getting the results you want. If you want to run, keep this principle foremost in your mind: *the more intense the exercise, the more you should emphasize your lazy way.* It would be best to do the K session of **WALKING/RUNNING** & **LOVING IT** before starting the **RUNNING** & **LOVING IT.**

Let's Talk About Running

There seems to be an inherent relationship between running and competition. Many people who begin running for fitness decide to run competitively. I have known several people who have started with fitness jogging, then trained for and completed a marathon. Then, their next step was to quit running and never again start. Years later, their fitness level is no better than it was before they started jogging for fitness.

To be clear, I have a great deal of appreciation for the accomplishments of the people I just referenced. I appreciate excellence in any form of human achievement and completing a marathon is certainly a significant human achievement. More specifically, completing a marathon is a significant *athletic* achievement.

It is also obvious that exercise carried to the extreme, e.g. competitive *workouts,* is critical to success in athletics. I marvel at the abilities of world class athletes and stand and cheer when I witness their feats. I nearly puke just *thinking* about the competitive workouts necessary for them to become world class athletes.

The point I want to make clear is this: *the concepts of fitness and competitive conditioning have* **nothing** *in common.* It might be argued that both involve exercise but the attitude and approach to exercise in a fitness program is fundamentally different than in a competitive conditioning program. The difference is so great that applying the word *exercise* to one concept should preclude its application to the other.

The self satisfaction and enhanced self image resulting from an achievement like completing a marathon has tremendous value. However, I'm convinced that the self satisfaction and enhanced self image resulting from living your life at an optimal fitness level is of ***greater*** value.

A lifetime of consistently and persistently doing a leisurely 20-minute running session is better than running a marathon.

And it's much lazier.

I am not trying to talk anyone out of running a marathon, especially since most have never considered it anyhow. I just know that running tends to stimulate one's competitive impulses. I want you to avoid the competitive attitude (law two of LAWS of EXERCISING & LOVING IT) and embrace your lazy way.

If you do run a marathon, you have my appreciation and congratulations - especially if you get back to your lazy way. Rather than becoming burned out of shape by the competitive conditioning necessary for your marathon, return to your lazy way. That way you can bask in the success of a glorious physical, mental, and emotional achievement and still live the rest of your life at optimal fitness level - and loving it!

Getting Older?

Be assured that I feel positive about running. However, without being negative, I believe a word of caution is required.

If you are beginning to feel a bit older and have no significant background with running, you need to be very careful. As one ages, it takes longer to recuperate from minor injuries that can result from doing too much too soon. Your younger self might recover from such injuries in a few days or weeks but as you get older those injuries can plague you for months or even years. In the worst cases, these problems can become chronic.

Make it a habit to review the LAWS of EXERCISING & LOVING IT and make sure you obey them. Failure to do so can result in punishment decreed by the natural state of the universe. Such punishment is immediate, automatic, and severe.

Rather than being negative, I am simply being lazy. In the context of this book's philosophy lazy is positive. If you want to run, whatever your age, do so in a lazy fashion. Develop your optimal performance level lazily and running can be part, or nearly all, of your optimal fitness level. Use you lazy way and running will make you feel *younger*.

Developing a 20-Minute Run

The K Session of the Walking/Running Program is five sets of six minutes for a total Session of thirty minutes. Each set is a four-minute walking interval followed by a two-minute running interval. Be sure you can do this before starting the running program.

This program is designed to develop a continuous 20-minute run. As before, use four sets of five minutes for your running sessions. For your first session try walking 3½ minutes followed by 1½ minutes of running (a five-minute set). Repeat this four times for your 20-minute session.

In succeeding sessions, stay with these interval times until you are completely comfortable changing them. Then gradually increase the running time while reducing the walking time. The idea is to cut a few seconds from each walking interval while adding that same number of seconds to the running interval.

Whenever you change interval times, do so by five seconds or less. If you start with 03:30 walking and 01:30 running, try 03:25 and 01:35 in each of your four, five-minute sets. Remember that you are you are decreasing the recuperation time you get from walking as you increase your running interval.

Even if you are young and in good shape, start with no more than 1½ minute running intervals and take several months to eliminate all the walking. There is no advantage to rushing. There is every advantage to moving consistently, persistently, and *very gradually* from your first through each successive session. Be lazy.

Keep in mind that any combination of walking and running times might be appropriate for your optimal session. You might find that you don't need a continuous 20-minute run. Be sure that your optimal session feels lazy.

Begin running your lazy way with two to five sessions per week. Allow yourself at least two recuperation days a week.

After you have done a 20-minute session of continuous running, you might want to check your distance. It's easy if you have access to a quarter mile track. Check your local junior highs, high schools, or colleges. You need only to count the number of ¼ mile laps you do in one session, and then divide by four.

You might also want to check your speed. The number of laps you complete on a ¼ mile track in 15 minutes equals the number of miles per hour you are running - i.e., six laps in 15 minutes is six mph; seven laps is seven mph; eight laps is eight mph.

If you are running two miles or less in 20 minutes, that is good! If you find it lazy to do two miles in 20 minutes, fine. To run faster or farther is moving into the competitive arena. Two miles, or *less,* in 20 minutes should provide an optimal running session. Experiment with the number of sessions per week to determine your optimal performance level.

<u>Reverse-goal:</u> Run two miles or less, and no longer than 20 minutes, in each running session.

I quit running competitively more than 50 years ago. I was so competitive that I burned myself out at age 14. Don't burn yourself out. Stay lazy and stay in great shape!

Coaching tip 8: Last fall, at age 68, I tried this lazy approach to developing a 20-minute run. I had started with 1½ minute walking intervals and 3½ minute running intervals. From late August to Early November, I had changed my interval times to 2½ minutes each and had run this session several times. Even being extremely lazy, *I broke my damned old knee!* I'm telling you, be lazy. Don't try hard or push yourself at all!

Stretching & Logging for Running Your Lazy Way

As before, cool down and stretch for at least five minutes after finishing a session. Do stretching exercises one, two, three, and four from **STRETCHING & LOVING** IT during the cooling down period following each   session.

Date	Sets	Minutes Minutes Walking Runnings	Total Walk	Total Run
11/21	4	1:30 + 3:30	6:00	14:00

The sample log shows four sets of 1½ minute walks plus 3½ minute runs. This session was performed on November 21. It provided six minutes of walking and fourteen minutes of running.

If you are doing a 20-minute run with no intervals, your log can be very simple. A check mark on a calendar date might be sufficient. It's simple, but this log is also very important. It gives quick visual verification of your consistency and persistence. It encourages you continuously by substantiating your great shape.

Date	Distance	Rate
11/21	2 miles	6 mph

If you prefer to include your distance and/or speed in your log, you can use this example. If you know your distance for a 20-minute run, you need only multiply the distance by three to get your running speed in miles per hour.

SWIMMING & LOVING IT

If you haven't learned to swim, you should learn. Call your local Red Cross or your high school's swimming coach and ask for a "learn to swim" program for adults. Why? - because water's natural buoyancy makes it an ideal venue for the lazy way approach to exercise. Buoyancy eliminates undue physical stress to muscles and joints during your swimming sessions.

The difficulty in exercising on dry land, beyond the physical exertion for exercising, is the additional work needed for overcoming gravity. On land your muscles and joints must constantly work to overcome gravity.

Water pampers your muscles and joints by supporting them against gravity. In water, your joints need to manage only the forces from muscular effort.

Your muscles exert only the forces necessary for propulsion.

The reduced stress on your muscles and joints allows you to swim much farther than you would probably expect - especially if you use your lazy way. Because swimming treats your body with kid gloves, I can make this prediction: *you can swim 800 yards without stopping.*

I'm not trying to give you a goal to seek. I'm just noting that you already have that capacity. In fact, you can swim 800 yards lazily - and loving it.

That's worth repeating. If you can swim, or when you learn to swim, you can swim 800 yards without stopping.

Because you have the innate capacity to swim 800 yards, it is not necessary to set this as a goal. Besides, you should avoid setting goals for fitness sessions (law four from **LAWS** of **EXERCISING** & **LOVING IT).**

The obvious first step - especially if you don't know how to swim - is to learn. Call a Red Cross chapter or the closest high school swimming coach and ask about adult learn to swim programs.

If you can swim, look for a place where you can exercise three or more times a week throughout the year. Local high schools or colleges are good starting points. Many often allow community access to their pools. A pool of 20 yards or longer is better but use smaller pools if that's all that's available.

Start your program with the crawl stroke. With your body prone in the water, use a flutter kick. Alternate the arms in the stroke, breathing to the side. Don't worry about form or how you look. You are being lazy and not competitive. Your stroke mechanics will improve as you continue and even if they don't, you can still get into great shape.

Find a sporting goods store and buy a good pair of goggles. You probably won't want to swim with your eyes shut, and it can be uncomfortable to swim with your eyes open and without goggles.

Your First Continuous 400 Yard Swim

Start on a small scale - swim one length of the pool, regardless of the distance. Emphasize the arm pull rather than the leg kick. Stop after the first length and rest until you are ready to swim back.

Don't be too hasty to resume swimming immediately. You should be completely ready, both physically and emotionally. If one length is too far, swim alongside a wall, stopping for a rest in the middle. You can also walk on the bottom of the pool until you are ready to continue. Continue with your swim only when you feel ready to do so.

As you swim, continue resting whenever needed for as long as necessary. Swim no farther than one length before resting. Stay in your session until you have completed about 400 yards. This is 16 lengths of a 25-yard pool, 20 lengths of a 20-yard pool, or about eight lengths of a 50-meter pool. For shorter pools, estimate their lengths. Your best estimate is good enough.

This type of swim could take from 15 minutes to over an hour, depending on your speed and length of time that you rest. Pay no attention to time. Avoid pushing yourself and take all the time you need. Be lazy.

When you can do 400 yards one length at a time with untimed intervals, time the rest interval after your first length. That can serve as the rest interval after each length for the remainder of your swim. Example: you measure 90 seconds as the time of the interval after your first length. So, you do one length, rest 90 seconds; a second length, again rest 90 seconds; a third length, rest another 90 seconds. The idea is to repeat the process until you complete the number of lengths that equals 400 yards.

In subsequent sessions cut your rest interval time gradually. You can set your rest interval times based on how you *feel.* Feel lazy. Each cut from your rest intervals should be from one to ten seconds. Take as many sessions as necessary to lower your intervals to 30 seconds. Stay lazy.

When you are resting no more than 30 seconds between single lengths, and your total time in the session is no more than 25 minutes, increase your endurance by doing two lengths at a time. After two lengths without stopping, rest as necessary before doing two more. When you can swim 400 yards two lengths at a time using untimed rest periods, you again time your first rest interval. Then, as you did before, slowly lessen the timed intervals down to 30 seconds.

Now you begin doing the 400 yards four lengths at a time before resting. Use the same planned sequence as with your one and two length-at-a-time sessions ... 1) start with untimed intervals between four-length swims, 2) time your first interval to determine your interval times, 3) gradually reduce your interval times down to 30 seconds.

Next, begin doing eight continuous lengths before resting. If you do eight lengths in a 50-meter pool you are swimming 400 meters. In a 25-yard pool, you use another untimed rest period and then do a second eight lengths. When you can complete the second eight lengths continuously, time your rest- interval. Then lazily decrease the interval until you are doing 16 lengths (400 yards) nonstop.

Stretching for Swimming & Loving It

Do stretching exercise five from **STRETCHING** & **LOVING IT** while drying with a towel after each lazy swimming   session.

Your Second 400 Yard Swim

Your 400-yard swim becomes your regular swimming session until you feel you want and are ready to tackle more exercise. After doing 400-yard sessions for a while, you will feel ready to add a second 400-yards to your session. At that point, you rest until you feel completely recuperated. Then start your second 400 and see how it goes. You might be surprised that you can easily do the second 400 without stopping.

Remember, completing the second 400 without stopping is not a goal. Do *not* do the second 400 continuously unless you feel lazy for the entire distance. Stop at any point during the process. Stay lazy. If you do the second 400 lazily, time the interval between your 400's. Then, in successive sessions, gradually reduce your interval to zero. Now you are doing a continuous 800-yard swim. See, I told you so!

If you don't finish your second 400 lazily on your first try, you already have a simple alternative. You only need to do your first 400, rest as needed, then implement the same plan you used in the section **Your First Continuous 400 Yard Swim.** Adapt the first plan in any ways that are comfortable, lazy and allow you to apply your preferred pace. You will find that it will be easier and takes fewer sessions to do your second 400 continuously than it was for your first 400.

Use untimed rest periods after your first 400 until you can comfortably do a continuous second 400. After you do an uninterrupted second 400, time your rest interval between the two 400s. Then slowly and lazily eliminate your interval over an unplanned number of subsequent sessions.

An 800-yard untimed swim might provide your optimal swimming session. If you feel you need more exercise, go for it by timing your swim. Gradually increase your speed, lowering your time for 800 yards, until you have an optimal session. Once your sessions are optimal, you can experiment with the number of swims per week needed for your optimal performance level.

Reverse-goals: if you are by nature an inveterate goal-setter, here are a couple of objectives that should be easy to follow:

1. Avoid swimming faster than 16 minutes for 800 yards. Faster swimming is becoming competitive. Be lazy and stay in permanent great shape.
2. Pledge on the family Bible that you will not attempt to swim the English Channel.

Alternating two or three swims with two or three walks or runs per week is a terrific cardiorespiratory fitness program. The combination of swimming with either walking or running builds strength and endurance in nearly all the large muscles of your body.

Your swimming program will give you more pleasure as you become more efficient and learn more about what you are doing. A good way to do both is to read any good book on swimming for fitness.

Should you choose that path, keep firmly in mind that most, if not all, of the authors of these books are *very* competitive. Their competitiveness is why they thoroughly understand topics such as stroke mechanics and how to combat "swimmer's ear." Use their considerable and valuable knowledge to your advantage. But rather than becoming competitive, remember your lazy way.

Logging for Swimming & Loving It

Usually, you will find it more convenient to log your swims after showering, drying, and dressing. However, don't wait too long to put the record on paper. You should mark your logs immediately following your sessions. I suggest carrying a purse/shirt-pocket size notebook to the locker. Be sure to remember a pencil or pen.

When you are doing an 800-yard swim, you need only to note your date and time. The more sessions you add to your log the more comfortable and encouraged you become with **SWIMMING** & **LOVING** IT.

Sample Swimming Log					
Date	Lengths per Set	# Sets	Rest Interval	Session Time	Distance
1/27/22	1	8	Untimed	23 mins	200 yards

Enjoying Swimming & Loving It

Unlike many "ground-based" exercises, it is difficult to utilize external input (listening to music, watching a television program) to enjoy your swimming sessions. You really don't need it. Swimming is a very enjoyable activity in and of itself. It is especially enjoyable when you use your lazy way.

If you must have a diversion, plan on rewarding yourself *immediately after* your swim. Examples: time your session to allow enough time afterward to relax in a hot tub or get to a theater just before the movie begins. Or meet a friend for lunch. Allocate the time immediately following your session for something you enjoy. Relate your swims to something you always enjoy, and your swims automatically become more fun.

Remember, the idea is to change your lifestyle, not to accomplish a goal. The more fun you have, the lazier you feel - and vice versa! This approach makes for an easy, pleasant way to change your lifestyle.

STRENGTH TRAINING & LOVING IT

Strength training is the best value you can get from exercise. It provides great benefits with a minimum of time or effort. The extra energy you feel from simply being able to move your body around more easily makes it a great activity.

Another bonus is that the improved tone of your muscles improves your appearance dramatically. If you want to look good on the beach, adding strength training to your aerobics program is an integral part of your preferred optimal fitness program. While strength training is not necessarily the best method of weight reduction, it represents an ideal method for improving your appearance - *fat* reduction.

Immediate Success

Increasing the strength of your muscles is quick and easy! This isn't hype or sales copy. (Would I be trying to sell you a book you are already reading?) If you have no prior experience with strength training, your first session can increase your strength by 15% to 25%. I know this because in an earlier life I wrote weight training programs for new health club members. I would instruct them to do two sets of 15 reps for a first workout. When they progressed to the next workout, using the same set of weights, they could usually do 20 reps for their first set and still do 17 or 18 reps on the second. That's a 25% increase in strength in one session. If they preferred increasing the weights, rather than the number of reps, they could generally increase their weights by 15%-25% and still do both sets of 15 reps.

While these new members were able to continue increasing their strength, measurable gains immediately became slower and more difficult to achieve. Sessions would tend to become more intense making them more arduous - and less enjoyable. Progressively greater intensity would cause increases in strength; but the payoff in strength increases would become less and less compared to the continuously increasing effort required. Eventually - usually long before their first-year memberships expired - the extra effort would become too great for the limited additional reward.

That first big increase was always exciting and encouraging. But as the workload increased, excitement waned, and encouragement became minimal. As is usually *still* the norm, competitive conditioning continued to be promoted. The joy of a session turned to drudgery. Burn-out then ensued.

Many years ago, I began to think it would be worthwhile to simply continue doing the very easy *second* workout - immediate success, lots of benefit, little effort. My mind was slowly beginning to formulate your lazy way to great shape.

Competitive Weight Training?

Weight training is much like running ... it can stimulate competition. Bring a new guy into a gym and the first thing he will want to do is see how much he can lift.

If he trains by himself, he will keep competing against himself, trying to add more and more weight until it is too hard to do. When it gets too hard, he will get discouraged. He might fight to stay with it for a while, but he will eventually quit.

If two guys share a space for doing a bench press in a noncompetitive "fitness" workout, there is a 100% probability that both will notice who lifts the most weight. There is a nearly equal probability that the one who lifts the most will feel superior, while he who lifts least will feel inferior. Regarding their fitness levels, both attitudes are utterly inaccurate and totally irrelevant.

Having established who is "best," they might not continue to compete against each other. But each individual will continue to compete against himself. They will continue working hard in subsequent workouts until they quit. Both will probably quit early on because competitive conditioning is just too difficult. The result is that they will lose whatever gains they made.

There may be a non-competitive lazy way to use weights for strength training, but I suggest you use the following simple, easy to use, and inexpensive alternative. This alternative provides strength training your lazy way.

Your Lazy Way to Strength

Rubber stretch cords are great tools to substitute for weights. It is difficult to measure the amount of resistance you are using with a stretch cord, but that's a good thing. Since you don't know how much resistance you are using, it is difficult to compete, even against yourself. This allows you to exercise for the value of the exercise rather than to achieve an artificial goal.

These cords are lightweight and take up very little space which makes them convenient for carrying, traveling, and storing. They can be as effective as weights for increasing tone, improving shape, and building strength.

Safety

With several precautions, stretch cords are safe to use. Possible problems might be having one break during an exercise or to slip from a point of attachment. The simple safeguards are to check the cord for flaws which might cause it to break and be sure they are safely attached. Even then little could go wrong other than getting slapped by an end of the broken cord.

To be fair and speaking from experience, this can hurt! In the event the cord breaks or breaks loose, you do not want it to strike you or anyone else. Be sure nobody is close enough to get slapped.

In most exercises, you will be pushing or pulling the cord in directions away from your body. Be sure you are not doing something that could cause a broken cord to strike you. Be certain that you can't be struck in the head. Observe these simple precautions, and you should never have any problems. In the last thirty years, I've only been slapped by a broken cord once. But, yeah, it hurt- and it won't happen to me again.

The latex tubing used in hospitals can serve as great stretch cords for exercise. Though not made for exercise, latex tubing may be the best dollar value of anything you can buy for exercise. I use tubing with 31s" outside diameter, ¼" inside diameter, and 11/16" walls. The tubing might be available in stores that sell equipment and supplies to hospitals, physicians, and surgeons. Check the phone book under: 1) hospital equipment and supplies, 2) physicians and surgeons' equipment and supplies, 3) medical supplies.

Another resource could be in the plumbing departments of the big retail home improvement stores. A 10' length should serve your purpose. If you can't find a retail outlet for it, or if it is more convenient to order from https://ExercisingAndLovingIt.com by mail.

You can also do an Internet search and find sets with colored cords of different resistance. They come with build in handles and a way to attach to the inside of a closed-door frame.

Your Stretch Cord Sessions

Before each exercise, take up any slack in the cord. Try 20 repetitions of an exercise in the first session and stop if you begin to tire before going on to another 20 reps. After the first session, adjust the tension in the cord so your muscles feel exercised after 20 reps. Do 20 reps per exercise per session. You will grow stronger from doing these sessions.

Be lazy. Avoid exhausting your muscles and don't force strength increases. Always feel like you can do several more reps at the end of a set. Do about 75-80% of your maximum capacity. For instance, if 25 reps are the most you can do you, do no more than 20. If you do 15, and feel like you could just *barely* finish 20, stop at 15 or 16. If 10 are the most you can do, do eight or less.

If you stay lazy, you will likely become strong enough to easily increase the cord's tension in subsequent sessions. You might also decide to use more than one strand of the cord for some exercises. Increase the cord's tension only because you will feel *too* lazy if you don't.

Reject any impulse to push yourself to increase the tension in the cord. Pushing yourself won't make you any stronger than being lazy and consistent. So, if you stay lazy you will become just as strong; and, you'll stay strong because you won't burn out.

Twenty reps/set will exercise the muscles sufficiently in each session. Do one set of 20-reps of each of the exercises you use, and you can complete your sessions in less than 15 minutes. You can do your session nearly everyday, and you should do it at least three times a week. For a strength program, less than 15 minutes per session is unprecedented laziness. Yet you will experience noticeable and significant results. Like I said, this is your lazy way to great shape.

If you consistently use the same exercises in your sessions, you can simply log dates of your sessions with checkmarks to show sessions were complete. Then you only note changes you make in the exercises. Use music, television, or other passive entertainment to make your sessions more enjoyable.

Your Stretch Cord Exercises

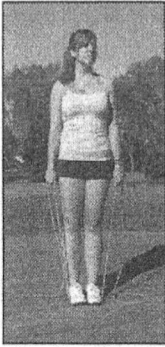 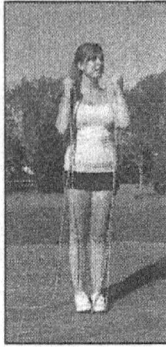 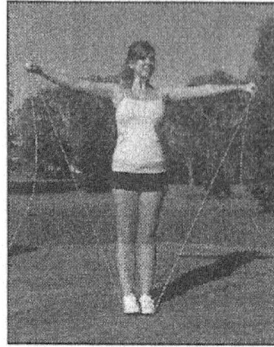 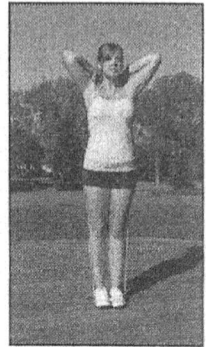

Starting Pos   Picture 1   Picture 2   Picture 3a

Exercises 1, 2, 3

1. Keep your elbows at your sides and pull your hands up to your shoulders. Allow your elbows to come slightly forward to bring your hands as close a possible to your shoulders (picture 1). Lower your hands to starting position for one rep.

2. Lift your arms sideward, elbows straight until your hands reach the height of your ears (picture 2). Lower your hands to starting position for one rep.

3. Raise your hands to your shoulders and place your elbows inside and forward of the cord. Move the cord around back of you then point your elbows upward (picture 3a).

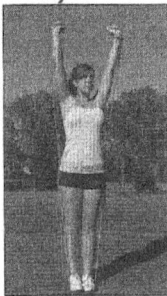 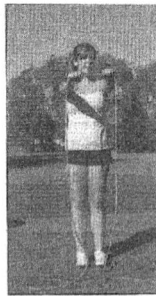 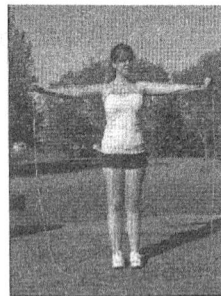

Picture 3b   Picture 4a   Picture 4b

94

This is a new starting position for the exercise. Keep your elbows in place and extend your arms till they point straight up (picture 3b). Then **lower** your arms to starting position (also, picture 3a) for one rep.

4. Stand, arms extended forward parallel to the floor holding the cord in each hand. Begin with your hands apart about shoulder width (picture 4a). Keep your elbows straight and pull your arms sideward as far as you can (picture 4b). Keep your arms parallel to the floor as you pull. Return to starting position for one rep.

5. Place your cord around the hinged edge of a door. Stand with your back against the other edge holding the cord in each hand.

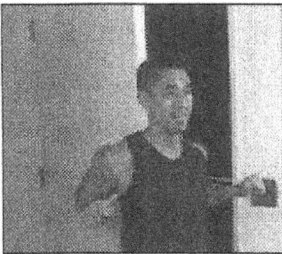 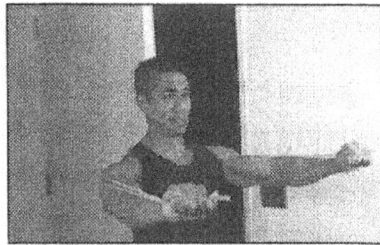

Picture 5a   Picture 5b

Begin with your hands close to your shoulders and your elbows pointed to the rear (picture 5a). Push your hands forward stretching the cord until your elbows are straight (picture 5b).

Return your hands and arms to starting position for one rep.

6. Stand facing the edge of the door and place the cord over the top of the door. Hold the cord in each hand with your arms extended sideward, elbows straight, and hands higher than your head. Keep your elbows straight

and pull your hands sideward and down as far as possible (Picture 6). Raise your hands to starting position for one rep.

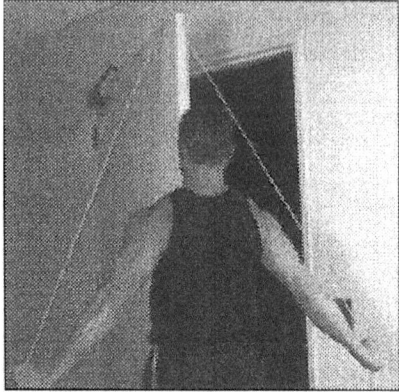
Picture 6

7. Sit on the floor, legs straight. Grip the ends of the cord in each hand and place the middle of the cord around the arches of your feet (picture 7a). Keep your body upright and pull and your hands to your chest (picture 7b). Return to starting position for one rep.

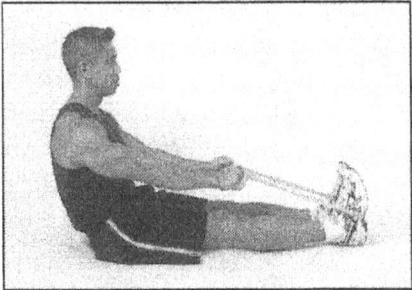
Picture 7a

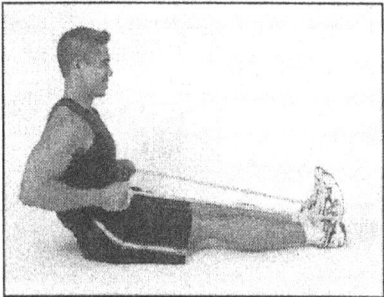
Picture 7b

8. Wrap the middle of the cord around one leg just above the knee. Place the ends of the cord around a doorknob. Hold the two ends in one hand and move away from the doorknob until the cord pulls your leg to about a $45°$ angle from your body (picture 8a).

Support your balance with your other hand on some stable object. Keep your leg straight and pull your foot toward your support foot till your feet touch (picture 8b). Return to starting position for one rep.

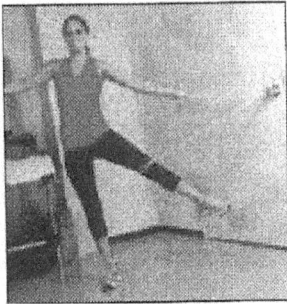

Picture 8a

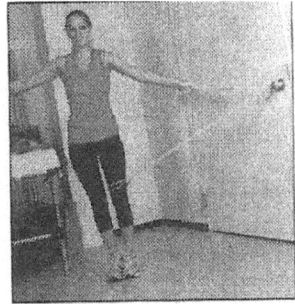

Picture 8b

9. Stand nextto a support object, feet shoulder width apart. Wrap the cord around the middle of one leg just above the knee. Wrap the cord around the other leg at the same point just above the knee. Wrap both ends of the cord around a doorknob. Then hold the doorknob to keep the ends in place and to support your balance. Pull the exercising leg sideward and upward to about a 45 angle from your body (picture 9). Return to starting position for one rep.

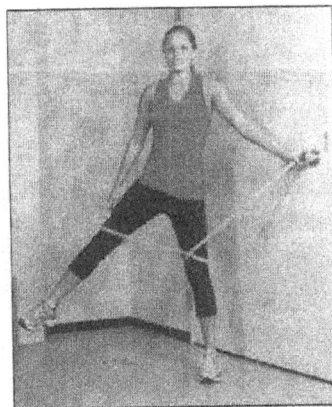

Picture 9

STRETCHING & LOVING IT

Stretching: 1) makes it easier to do your other lazy way programs, 2) prevents or reduces muscle soreness, 3) helps to prevent and/or reduce the severity of injuries from exercising, 4) keeps your joints flexible and your muscles supple.

The muscles of the arms or legs tend to tighten because they are seldom used through their entire range of motion. Stretching the muscles through their full range helps to compensate for this. The exercises should be performed during your cooling down period after your exercise sessions.

This simple program is not designed to dramatically increase joint flexibility and range of motion. If you wish to increase the flexibility and range of motion of your body's joints, you should consider more thorough stretching programs. If you are interested in stretching as a stand-alone fitness program, check appropriate sources in your library or talk to a physical therapist.

Your Stretching Exercises

1. Many of the exercises designed to stretch your thigh muscles place excessive stress on your knees or lower back. This exercise provides stretching for your thighs while avoiding knee and back problems.

Place the toes and instep of one back foot on top of a desk, chair, or some other stable object. The object should be about as high as your hips. Stand far enough away from the object that the long muscles in front of

your elevated thigh feel stretched. Gently bend the knee
of the support leg to stretch your thigh muscles further

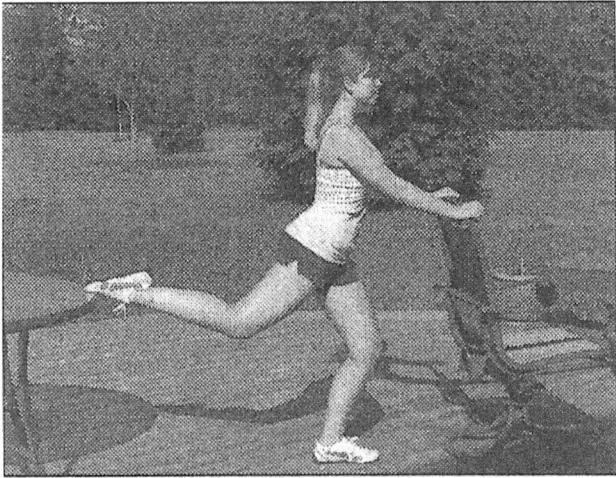

Exercise 1

(pictured). Maintain your position, relax then straighten
your elevated knee to increase the stretch. You can also
arch your back, bend your knees, and use movements
from your pelvis to gain more stretch. At each knee move
your pelvis and your lower back until you feel the muscles
and joints are stretched to the limit. Hold this final
stretched position for six seconds. Repeat the exercise
with the other leg.

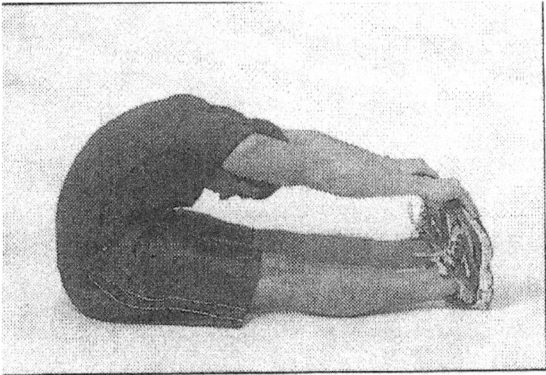

Exercise 2

2. Sit on the floor legs straight and together. Keep your legs straight, slowly, and gently lean forward moving your nose toward your knees. You will feel the stretch behind your knees and along the back of your upper legs (hamstrings). You might feel significant stretch along your spine. When you reach your limit, hold the stretched position, and relax.   Then gently attempt to increase the stretch. Hold the increased stretch position and again relax. Repeat, continuing to increase the stretch, then holding and relaxing until you feel you have reached your maximum stretch (pictured). Hold that stretch for six seconds.

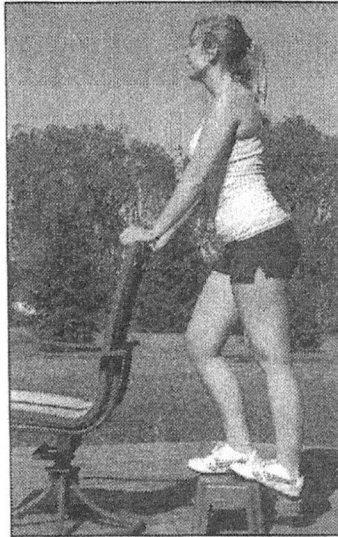

Exercise 3

3. Stand with the ball of your left foot on a stair step or some other platform. Place all of the right foot on the platform for balance. Keep your left leg straight and lower your left heel below the level of the platform stretching the calf of your left leg. There are three ways to increase your calf s stretch: 1) drive your left

heel lower, 2) transfer weight from your right leg to the ball of your left foot, 3) keep your left knee straight and lean forward from your left ankle. When you reach your limit, hold the stretched position, and relax. Then try **Exercise 3** to increase the stretch by the three listed methods. Repeat until you feel you have reached your maximum stretch (pictured). Hold your maximum stretch for six seconds. Repeat the exercise stretching the right calf.

4. This exercise stretches the soleus muscle below your calf. This is the same as exercise three with one change. Bend the knee above your stretching calf to about 45° (pictured). Then use the three ways you stretched your calf in the third exercise to stretch the muscle below your calf. Stretch the muscles on both the left and right sides.

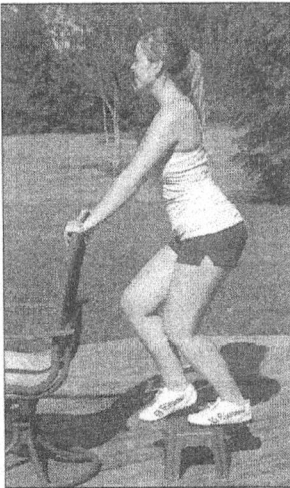

Exercise 4

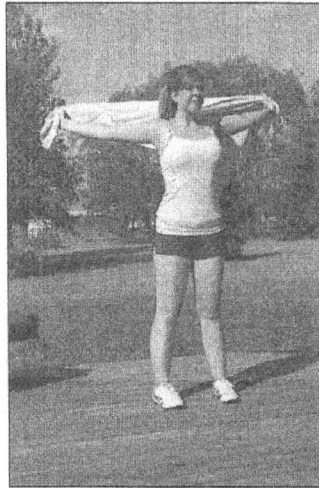

Exercise 5

5. This exercise is great to do when you are drying off after a shower or bath. One reason is because the warmth of the water helps loosen your

joints. The other is that you can use a towel as the aid to do the exercise. This stretch is a worthy addition to your exercise, but it is unnecessary as part of the cool-down for other exercise sessions. Get in the habit of doing it every time you dry off.

Hold the ends of a towel in each hand. Raise the towel above your head. Keep your elbows straight and try to bring the towel down **behind** you. You will feel the stretch in your shoulders and possibly across your chest. If you cannot bring the towel all the way down, either find a longer towel or bend one elbow while keeping the other elbow straight.

Adjust the tension in the towel by gripping it with your hands closer together or farther apart. Lower both arms at the same time. Lower the towel to your back adjusting the tension to **just** barely lower it down. At this **point**, optimal stretch (exercise 5, p 101), gently move the towel down past the maximum stretch point then up again. Repeat this movement until you feel your shoulder joints are thoroughly stretched.

It isn't necessary to **log** your stretching sessions **because** some stretching should be included in all your sessions.

Your lazy way to great shape can be applied to *any* exercise activity. If you need **help** in applying these principles to a specific activity, contact me at <u>https://ExercisingAndLovingIt.com</u>. Or write and identify yourself as a reader of this book and I will reply.

AFTERWORD

You may be aware that I am not a newcomer to the discipline of adult fitness. My first writing on fitness was more than 35 years ago. I have been in and out of this business ever since. I have become neither rich nor famous, although I have had short flirtations with both (rich is better than famous).

Two principles have become evident over these years. First, the attitudes and philosophy of fitness expressed in the preceding pages present, by far, the most successful methodology for achieving and maintaining lifetime fitness. Second, fitness is a lifestyle. It is not a program. It is not a fad. Neither is it a 10-day diet, nor the successful completion of a triathlon. If it is anything less than a lifestyle, it is not fitness.

The reason I am so sure of the first principle is the success of my first book, *How to Flatten Your Stomach.* I have no idea where that title came from, but it was a great title. It seemed - still seems - like a gift from the universe. Great titles, like great covers, sell books. However, great books are irrespective of their titles or covers. To this day, I have people seeking me out to replace copies of that little book they purchased decades ago. These people no longer care about the title that sold them the book. They love the *program.*

I didn't fully understand the philosophy of *Your Lazy Way to Great Shape* when I wrote my first book. But I was beginning to "feel" it. While not overtly expressed, the lazy way philosophy influenced my writing. I am convinced this philosophy is the reason *How to Flatten Your Stomach* was a successful program, not just a successful sale. That success has convinced me of the truth of the first principle - the lazy way is the best way to be fit for life.

That second principle, that fitness is a lifestyle, is more complicated. I have always believed that fitness is a way of life. However, I wasn't sufficiently focused on that idea. There is a significant difference between believing and understanding. I didn't *understand* this principle until sometime after November 2008. At that time, I was diagnosed as pre-diabetic. After learning of the medical disasters that can be caused by diabetes, I was terrified.

I knew that I had to be consistent and persistent with sufficient exercise to control my blood glucose, or else I would pay dearly. An on-again/off-again fitness program would not suffice. For me, fitness *had* to be a way of life. I knew that if I pushed myself or tried too hard, I'd burn out. I knew that if I exercised as I did when I was a competitive athlete, or with that competitive attitude, there would be "off seasons" - periodic quitting! I know what likely awaits me if I ever quit.

I had, of course, been preaching the importance and correctness of these "lazy" techniques for years. But this time I had to take my own advice. I did. It worked. I no longer simply believe that fitness is a way of life. That second principle is now firmly entrenched in my mind. I am thoroughly focused on it. I *understand* that fitness is a way of life.

The good news is that fitness is a very good way of life. I have become convinced that the lifestyles of the rich and famous are inferior to the lifestyles of the fit and non-famous (unless maybe you are also rich, famous, and fit).

Three years ago, I was working very hard and not experiencing any enjoyment. I certainly was not healthy, productive or happy. I felt like I had come to a dead end and didn't much care about life. Thank God I was diagnosed as pre- diabetic.

Now, I am seriously lazy. And since I continually apply that sixth law from the **LAWS for EXERCISING and LOVING IT,** I actually do love exercising. At 68 when first published and now 79 for the second edition, I don't know how long I am going to live but I do know that I am looking forward to living. I am not the same person that I was four years ago. I no longer look, feel, think nor act the same. I am much healthier, more productive, and happier. My moods are better. I feel less stress.

I know that these exercise programs are the primary reasons for the improvements in my life. It makes me feel terrific that they are a permanent part of my life. After a lifetime of sports and training, this newfound understanding has revolutionized my lifestyle.

Because exercise must be a permanent part of your life, it makes no difference how long it takes to reach an optimal fitness level - great shape! You have the rest of your life! Just get started, keep going and you *are* in great shape. It is my fervent hope and sincere desire that you too are revolutionizing your lifestyle with the concept of *Exercising and Loving It.*

Jim Everroad October 29, 2012   First Edition,
            December 2, 2022 Second Edition

     Thank you very much for your interest in these programs, and in <u>Exercising & Loving It.</u> Please let me know what you think about this book. Tell me when you feel fit and are in great shape. When people start telling you how good you look, let me know that too.

     Send <u>https://ExercisingAndLovingIt.com</u> Your comments. Use the Contact Us form.

     Or mail to: Coach Jim Everroad, Everroad Publishing Company, 2211 Franklin Street, Columbus, IN 47201 USA

     I would love to hear from you.